T0219557

Paul Dugdale BMBS, MA, MPH, PhD, FAFPHM is a senior medical specialist in ACT Health where he is Director of Chronic Disease Management. From 2002 to 2007 he was the ACT Chief Health Officer and Executive Director of ACT Health's Population Health Division. He has been a member of the National Health and Medical Research Council and the Australian Council for Safety and Quality in Health Care. He worked previously in the Health Financing Division of the Commonwealth Department of Health and Aged Care, the Health Service Planning Division of NSW Health, was medical superintendent at The Liverpool Hospital (Sydney) and was private secretary to the Commonwealth Minister for Health Neal Blewett.

He is a Fellow of the Australasian Faculty of Public Health Medicine in the Royal Australasian College of Physicians, Associate Professor of Public Health in the Australian National University Medical School and Director of the ANU Centre for Health Stewardship.

Doing Health Policy in Australia

Paul Dugdale

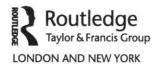

Routledge
Taylor & Francis Group

LONDON AND NEW YORK

First published 2008 by Allen & Unwin

Published 2020 by Routledge
2 Park Square, Milton Park, Abingdon, Oxon OX14 4RN
605 Third Avenue, New York, NY 10017

Routledge is an imprint of the Taylor & Francis Group, an informa business

National Library of Australia
Cataloguing-in-Publication entry:

Dugdale, Paul M.

Doing health policy in Australia

Includes index.
Bibliography.

Public health—Australia.
Medical policy—Australia.

362.10994

Index by Russell Brooks
Set in 11/14 pt Minion by Midland Typesetters, Australia

ISBN-13: 9781741753950 (pbk)

CONTENTS

ACKNOWLEDGMENTS

ACT Health has provided support and leave to complete this book. The Australian National University provided a place to write much of it. The National Health and Medical Research Council provided scholarship support for Chapters 3 to 6. The Australian Council for Safety and Quality in Health Care and the Australian Research Council each provided financial support for various parts of Chapter 7. Early versions of parts of Chapter 10 have been published by the *Australian Journal of Public Administration* (Dugdale 1991) and Allen & Unwin (Dugdale 1998). Thank you to Barry Hindess and Charles Kerr for helping me learn to think about the topics in this book, and to Robyn Penman for comments on the manuscript. This book draws on our family ethos of inquiry and public spiritedness for which I would like to thank my parents, my children and my wife, Alison Morehead. Here's to your health!

1.

THE HEALTH POLICY SCENE

A VIGOROUS CURIOSITY

Health policy is a big field. Most newspapers carry a story on it in every edition. Around one in ten people work in health, and one in every ten dollars spent in Australia is spent on health—the majority of it public money. During their working life, perhaps the majority of people who work in the health sector, and a good percentage of people who work in government policy more generally, will participate in formal health policy discussions. Most will draw on their own experience and general ideas of what should happen. Some will represent the experience and ideas of colleagues with whom they have discussed the issue. A small minority will participate as skilled policy analysts.

Much of the content of this book has been driven by curiosity about how the health system works. Dr Sid Sax's classic book on Australian health policy in the Medibank era, *A Strife of Interests* (Sax 1984), took its title from the late nineteenth century definition of politics in Ambrose Bierce's satirical *Devil's Dictionary* (Bierce 1967). Sax's basic proposition was that health policy could be understood as the playing out of the various interests involved, which could be seen by looking behind the masquerade of principles with which they disguised themselves. As Sax's life as a reformer and his published work demonstrate, curiosity about what drives reform of the health system finds more than the strife of interests. Personal or collective self-interest, the pursuit of freedom and happiness, public acclaim, humanism and the ethos of science all play a part. Curiously, humanitarian concern is perhaps the highest common factor amongst the variable self-interests in the equation (this alone justifies some suspicion about the nature of humanism). But humanitarian concerns don't seem to play a big part in setting the agenda for debate—in how some part or other of the health system becomes perceived as needing to be reformed, or change in some other part is considered off limits. Nor do they explain why some things can be done with widespread support and enthusiasm, and other things can only be done against enormous resistance.

There is also a curiosity about why the health system is the way it is, about the history of institutions and administrative arrangements that structure it. In particular, there is a curiosity about the history of the involvement of the state in health and reflection on the role of health in the constitution of the modern state. This is a curiosity about what is at the heart of various calls for reform, which can often be nutted out by careful thinking about what that aspect of the health system really does or what is really at stake in a reform proposal.

Australia's vigorous health policy scene is in rude health. To describe someone as being 'in rude health' gives an idea of inner vitality and strength, a capacity for doing hard work and taking vigorous pleasures, of robustness and a capacity to withstand the slings and arrows a broad exposure to life brings. We don't think of rude health as arising from careful dieting, a detailed exercise regime, regular medical surveillance and judicious choice of medications (preventive or otherwise). Rude health arises in some sense from the play of wildness in a suitable environment, rather than from judicious discipline and a detailed prescription. The health policy scene is like the talented school kid from a big country town offered a scholarship by the Australian Institute of Sport, rather than the sculpted athlete on the Olympic podium after long years of preparation.

The heterogeneity and vigour of health policy has been a longstanding feature of Australian civil society, and probably reflects the nature of our democratic-welfare-capitalist society on the one hand and the overall importance of health and health care on the other. The health systems that reflect our health policy have a few rough edges—perhaps quite a few—but mostly seem to work pretty well. Health outcomes for most of Australia's population are excellent, and health system performance is pretty good when measured in terms of value for money, quality of care and the match of health services with need. All of this can be improved on, of course, and there is a keen sense of this in health policy circles.

The health policy scene is vigorously populated by nine federal, state and territory governments, and scores of professional associations, charities and lobby groups. There are around 150 health and biotechnology companies listed on the Australian Stock Exchange. There is certainly no master plan, no readily identifiable dominant force in health policy since the relatively brief period during the making of Medicare by the federal government over 20 years ago. There has been a constant stream of reforms pursued at regional, state and national levels, some of which have created change and some not. New policy technologies and new programs turn up frequently and are only very occasionally self-evidently bad. Health policy-making is certainly somewhat unruly and debate is usually vigorous.

This book draws on social theory and history to explain some of the dynamics of the contemporary Australian health system. My hope in writing it is that it will be helpful for people working actively on reform of the health system, or studying to prepare themselves to work in health policy, management and reform. The sheer size of the health system, and its complexity, make it a difficult field to have a clear enough view to provide sound management, sensible policy and useful reform. One response to this complexity is to accumulate more and more knowledge about the system and its effects. While this is clearly a sensible approach, it is also important to think carefully about just what health is, what the health system is for, what its dynamics and tensions are and about the features of successful reform. This book addresses these types of questions. It draws on philosophical thought, political theory and the history of our current health system to reflect on why the health system is the way it is and on the sorts of strategies that work for managing and reforming it.

Many of my colleagues in the policy scene, if they read this book—and many of them read surprisingly broadly—will, I expect, find themselves arguing with my analysis on various topics. One of the key qualities of the policy generalist is that they are prepared to put down what they think or what they have gleaned about topics with which they are not overly familiar. In this book, I have written about things on which I have been involved in policy debate over the years—some more deeply than others, but each enough to offer some reflections on. I have little experience in Indigenous health policy, and so co-authored that chapter with Kerry Arabena, whose Indigenous health experience and analytical skills are highly sought after in the Australian policy scene.

Some sections of the book emphasise the history of how we came to take for granted the things that form the backdrop to a set of policy debates; other sections emphasise the detailed policy logic of a particular topic— perhaps relatively minor, but that illustrates the anxieties of the time. Much of the argument is presented in a fairly simple way, as opposed to the refined argument found in the peer-reviewed journals of the academy. I gloss over many things in an attempt to sketch some of the broad, muscular lines of argument. In a sense, it is the style of argument you might expect given my background as a health policy generalist in a big country town, having worked for governments of both persuasions.

This introductory chapter provides a summary of the main themes and an overview of each chapter in the book. The next two chapters discuss the nature of health and health policy. Chapters 4 and 5 discuss the history over the last few hundred years of three major features of the present health system: the medical profession; the hospital; and public health, in the sense of health protection and health promotion. The next two chapters are case studies of major reform efforts in the Australian health system, namely the creation of Medicare and the focus on safety and quality. The chapter on doing Indigenous health policy perhaps exhibits some frustration that successful major reform is yet to come. The chapter on health protection outlines some of the successes and challenges of mainstream public health practice. The book finishes with some reflections on consumer consultation and the ethics of policy activism within the health system.

In some ways, the question 'What is health?' has an intuitive answer that comes easily from the particular circumstance in which it is asked. However, like many of the other great questions—consider 'What is truth?'—the more deeply one thinks about it the less satisfactory the particular answers seem, and the best general answers come not as a precise, definitive statement but as part of a rich dialogue about the subject.

Chapter 2 takes this later tack in a definitional discussion of the nature of health. This chapter explains what we mean by health in everyday language and in what we call the health care system. It concludes with a discussion showing how population health can be situated at the centre of the development of contemporary society.

The United Nations has defined 'health' in the World Health Organization's constitution as follows: 'Health is a state of complete physical, mental and social well-being and not merely the absence of disease or infirmity' (WHO 1946). However, the actual meaning of both the term 'health' and the WHO definition remain enigmatic. This is more than a problem of language and more than a problem of historical context in the sense that only that which has no history is truly definable (Nietzsche 1969, p. 80).

Much health policy debate turns on the fact that health is always somewhat enigmatic: there is something about understanding it that always sits beyond clear conceptual grasp. Recognition of the enigmatic nature of health can help our analysis of the different perspectives that health professionals, their patients and the patients' carers all bring to specific episodes of health care provision, advice-giving or personal action for health. It also brings some insight into the endless innovation in health technology, systems of care and personal motivations directed towards being healthy or becoming healthier that characterise the health field. Furthermore, it helps us avoid errors that can result from using simplistic formulations of the meaning of health in designing health outcome measures in scientific studies.

HUMANISM AND HEALTH

Turning from a conceptual to an historical lens, health in society can be understood as the notion underpinning the development of the various health disciplines and systems in modernity (roughly the last 2000 years). Each of the disciplines of health—surgery, nursing, physiotherapy, public health and so on—has sought to create a field of science and a field of practice directed towards the betterment of Man. A glance at the historical idealism of the nineteenth century helps us understand the disciplinary structure of the health system as an historical expression of the notion of progress through knowledge, a concrete expression of the grand nineteenth century humanistic project suggested by the enlightenment of a hundred years earlier.

While this humanist perspective is still a common and powerful motivator of scientific, practical and policy endeavour in the health field, it is also helpful to come to grips with a broader analysis that gets outside of our desire to help or make progress and goes beyond the health field to show how population health can be situated at the centre of a broader social analysis. In this view, the issues that arise from the biological expansion of human populations are *the* central political and economic issues faced by modern societies in the medium- and long-term perspective. While this is just one scaffolding in the marketplace of social analysis, it is naturally suited to analysing health policy. I hope readers will find it provides some common ground across the seemingly disparate topics covered in subsequent chapters.

If the definition of health presents such a range of problems, it is not surprising that the idea of health policy also presents difficulties. However, it may be that the more enigmatic of these difficulties arise from the nature of health, and that the nature of policy relating to it can be analysed in a relatively straightforward way, using the analytical tools of (and subject to the limitations of) political and social theory. Whatever health itself may be, what is commonly called the health system is one of the great social machines of contemporary society. It is large and busy, with many moving parts, and it operates with a great deal of momentum. Many of those involved in it tinker with their parts and occasionally cooperate (perhaps unwittingly) in major changes. While health professionals and their patients are the main actors within the health machine, governments have the lead role in stewardship of the health system on behalf of the public.

Chapter 3 discusses general issues of health stewardship and public policy. It begins by considering what types of things the health departments of the Commonwealth, state and territory governments do, and examines the relationship between policy and research. It then provides a high-level overview of public sector funding for health and looks at how this is assembled with professional expertise and management structures to form the health system.

The activities of health departments in most western democracies are fundamentally related to the powers and responsibilities of the elected government—in Australia's case, the cabinet, including the health minister. Duly elected cabinet ministers are given executive commissions by the head of state—the state governors and the Governor-General—to operate the machinery of state. Health departments are the part of the machinery that works directly with the ministers for health to conceive and execute government policy. To do this, they formulate policy advice and execute government direction. Taking a somewhat simplistic view, the fields of policy action include: the structure of health systems and services; the regulation of health care activities; and health care financing by state treasuries and other means. Of course, these three fields interact—for example, in the heavy regulation of private insurance for health care.

Policy has a complex relationship to research. Contemporary policy-makers prefer to make policy based on sound research; publicly supported research is under pressure to contribute to the public good; and health systems strive to provide care supported by research. Yet the gulf remains between the world of the researcher and the world of the policy-maker or health service manager. There is no talking in the library and there are no books in the boardroom: research is an isolating activity whereas policy and management are subject to myriad pressures and demands. In such a context, it is useful to map out two major agendas: the major tasks facing health policy-makers and managers in relation to supporting and responding to health and medical research in Australia; and the way health and health systems researchers can support and be responsive to the reform efforts of health policy-makers and managers. These agendas have differences and overlaps. Research and stewardship align on some things and are unavoidably at odds on others. Understanding the relations between the two fields in a pragmatic way may help researchers avoid moralistic posturing and increase their contribution to research translation, relieve the exasperation of policy-makers and managers about the inadequacy of research, and perhaps even assist in their stewardship of the health research effort itself.

The chapter then turns to public financing of the health sector, which comprises around 10 per cent of total domestic economic activity in Australia. It encompasses many activities, institutions, agencies and companies. To make sense of this, it is useful to consider health systems as an assemblage of three main things: management, financing and expertise. These three things are knitted together at all levels of the health system and throughout our health services. Successful health care reform is always about creating new conjunctions of these three things, whether it be the revitalisation of a meandering community health service or the wholesale restructure of a state's regional health services.

This chapter begins an analysis of freedom in health policy that is developed in subsequent chapters. This ranges across classical economic ideas about freedom to practise linked to requirements for training and free markets with their limitations in health financing, to neo-liberal strategies such as publicly financed incentives for private medical practice and the politics of freedom that can be seen in the design and introduction of Medicare.

Chapter 4 recognises that almost all aspects of health stewardship require a dynamic understanding of the medical labour market. It provides a brief history of the development of licensing medical practitioners and other health professionals, and discusses how this licensing is controlled. It goes on to examine some of the major dynamics at play within the market for professional medical services by considering some of the incentives that influence doctors.

The government of medical practice couples the pastoral care relationship doctors have with their patients to the relationship between the state and a powerful group of its professional citizens. Legislatures in Australia started making laws in the late nineteenth century to register medical practitioners and to restrict the practice of medicine by others or to subordinate their practice to registered medical practitioners. This has been interpreted variously as a successful campaign for medical dominance or a classic example of liberal government through the creation of a self-governing sphere of civil society. Both these perspectives have currency within contemporary policy debates.

While financial incentives clearly affect the activities of doctors, this is powerfully modulated by the professional norms and organisational structures within which doctors work. This can clearly be seen in the operation of the Practice Incentives Program, a suite of incentives for general practitioners introduced around the turn of the millennium through the Memorandum of Understanding struck between the Australian government, the Royal Australian College of General Practitioners, Australian Divisions of General Practice and the Rural Doctors Association of Australia. This included incentives for accreditation, computerisation, care-planning, health assessments of the elderly, teaching medical students, practising in a rural area and cervical screening. Some of these incentives were associated with rapid increases in the relevant activity (e.g. accreditation, computerisation and student teaching) and some have had a slow or delayed effect on doctor activity that has been mediated by cultural and organisational change (e.g. care planning).

Chapter 5 turns from a professional perspective to an institutional perspective, and considers the development of public hospitals and public health. The institutional history of these has been fairly separate until the last couple of decades, but has now become entwined through the logic of population-based funding formulas and regionalisation of health service management.

The origins of modern clinical medicine lie in the seventeenth century turn in scientific practice towards detailed tabulation of observations as the principal way of understanding the world. By the beginning of the nineteenth century, teaching hospitals had been established for various health problems: maternity care, smallpox, fever, eye problems, and so on. By the beginning of the twentieth century, the current organisation of teaching hospitals into wards focused on the various organ systems had taken shape.

The origins of public health in the scientific era were oriented to the social body, rather than the internal workings of the individual body. William Petty's proposal to establish a statistical office in England and Leibniz's proposal to measure the power of a Prussian state through enumerating various characteristics of its population (Leibniz and Petty, quoted in Hacking 1990, p. 18) mark the beginning of the field of statistics ('state-istics'). Malthus published his essay on the principle of human population growth in the colonies in 1798 (Malthus 1970), and Chadwick produced a report in 1842 on the sanitary conditions of the working poor. This social concern for the health of the population combined in the nineteenth century with the emerging germ theory in the creation of a therapeutics of population health. The addition of the discipline of nosology—the taxonomy of diseases and causes of death—laid the basis for the powerful epidemiological techniques of the twentieth century.

The late twentieth century saw a conjunction of public health with hospital-based medicine, implicit in the emergence of the current dual meaning of public health in Australia (meaning health promotion and health protection efforts on the one hand, and the publicly funded health system on the other). With the advent of split purchaser provider structures, public health professionals found themselves blinking in the spotlight, called upon to advise about very large expenditures on tertiary hospital services. Although pure purchasing arrangements have gone out of fashion, population health thinking has continued to spread in hospital service development and reform.

THE MEDICARE ERA

Chapter 6 summarises the development of Medicare, Australia's national health scheme. After the Second World War, attempts by the Commonwealth Labor government to create a national health service similar to that in Britain were frustrated by political opposition and constitutional problems of federation, but resulted in the establishment of the

Pharmaceutical Benefits Scheme in 1948. Subsequently, the Menzies government established the Medical Benefits Scheme in 1954. To establish Medibank, the Whitlam government in 1974 entered into cost-sharing arrangements with the state governments to provide free universal access to public hospitals and nationalised insurance for medical services in 1975. This was to be financed by an income tax levy of 2 per cent, which the Opposition-controlled senate refused to pass, eventually precipitating the financial supply crisis and dismissal of the prime minister by the Governor-General. The succeeding Fraser government then set about dismantling Medibank and had substantially achieved this by 1981. The Hawke government once more contracted with the states for universal access to comprehensive hospital services and nationalised insurance for medical services in 1983 as part of the establishment of Medicare.

This development towards state financing of health care—which occurred throughout the OECD in the second half of the twentieth century—has been motivated by the increasing efficacy of expert medical interventions and the increasing difficulty consumers have in assessing their value. The nationalisation of insurance for medical services in the creation of the Medicare Benefits Scheme was perhaps the last national-isation of an industry in Australia, and is an interesting case study of the politics and mechanics of shifting health financing into the public sector.

With the intensification of government interest in health as the states and Commonwealth became involved in financing health care, the electoral politics of health were elaborated in more detail. The physicians' popu-lations were recognised as the politicians' electorates, and health care was elevated to a hip-pocket issue.

In a western democratic state such as Australia, policy debate and health system reform are threaded through and through with a concern for freedom of the public, health professionals and companies. Sometimes this concern is to restrict freedoms—for example, privacy laws that restrict the passing on of professionally acquired information about patients—and sometimes the concern is to preserve freedoms—for example, the way Medicare benefits effectively preserve the surgeon's ability to arrange treatment for their patients as the two of them see fit. Often, policies that provide freedoms to some types of actors in the health system necessarily place constraints on others. It could be said that the delineation of freedoms is one of the central necessities of health policy, and determines many of the ways in which health systems operate.

Chapter 7 turns to questions of the quality and safety of health care. Like many other industries, the health sector has taken up a range of continuous quality improvement activities. Review of adverse events by clinicians with their colleagues is a particularly important activity for clinicians striving to do no harm to patients. Analysis of these activities brings out some interesting features of the relationship between clinical freedom and corporate accountability for health professionals in publicly funded health care settings.

Building on the early work of the American time and motion analyst George Frederick Taylor (1911), the quality movement in post Second World War industrial society analysed industrial manufacturing operations as social systems. Technologies of quality improvement proliferated, initially in manufacturing but also in service industries as these grew in economic importance. These technologies included standards and accreditation, quality circles, continuous quality improvement and total quality management. These have all been adopted in various ways in health care. This has been driven by the financiers of health care—largely government and public administration in Australia. The same anxieties that drove governments to increase their role in financing health care have also driven government action to assure quality of care in general and safety of care in particular.

Financier, and thus management, interest in quality improvement supplemented the traditional professional activities of training and collegiality associated with medical licensing. Doctors have been somewhat difficult to engage in management-driven quality initiatives; however, the profession has developed its own contribution to quality improvement technology. As foreshadowed in Chapter 5, population health techniques have become part of the stock in trade of clinical management. Peer review and clinical audit, when they become more than just confessional, take the ethos and techniques of the clinical sciences from their traditional application in the scrutiny of beneficial therapies and apply them to the scrutiny of adverse events. Special legal protections that stop litigators and prosecutors accessing peer review and clinical audit material have been provided by legislatures to give courage to clinicians to participate in these activities.

The increasing scrutiny of adverse outcomes and mistakes requires an evolution in the makeup of what we might call the professional conscience, specifically a greater willingness to provide constructive criticism to one's colleagues and to engage institutional managers in clinical care. The struggle of clinicians for the freedom to act in their patients' best interests is transformed as they are drawn into giving accounts of the quality and safety of their clinical care to management. Conversely, corporate management is increasingly expected to ensure clinical governance is given as much attention as financial management. Regulation has played an important part in promoting quality and safety in health care. To work effectively, regulation must include ruinous powers to deal with recalcitrants. However, the bulk of quality and safety is driven by lower order regulatory approaches such as accreditation systems and creation of privileged forums for discussing error. Computerised information systems are playing an increasingly important role in advancing quality of care. As common standards for electronic communication and data-sharing are introduced, we should see the emergence of expert decision support systems that can provide the right guidance to the right clinicians at the time they are making decisions about the patient with them. Once this is a widespread reality, it could be seen as unsafe to provide clinical care without such electronic support.

Chapter 8, co-written with Kerry Arabena, considers how to do Indigenous health policy. We have to acknowledge at the outset that it could be done better than it has been. After considering the current context of Indigenous health policy and the value of consultation, we consider questions about whose idea of health should underpin health policy for Indigenous people. There is an important distinction between ideas of universalism in the health system and holism in health policy, with strengths and weaknesses in each approach. Universalism in health policy design can lead to poor access for Indigenous people. For example, the Medicare benefits system is designed in a way that means Indigenous people get proportionally fewer benefits from it than the members of the general population with similar health needs, because of the lack of doctors providing services to Indigenous people for which they could claim a benefit. On the other hand, a holistic approach is particularly important for addressing ill-health born of social problems and dislocations.

We then discuss some of the relations of art to health policy, drawing on Kerry Arabena's experience in the Western Desert, where she used art as a creative means of engagement and to enable the expression of ideas about health. In an interesting twist, art has also provided the Pintubi people with the economic means to establish a renal dialysis unit that has enabled their elders to return to their homeland, one of the most geographically isolated communities on the planet. The chapter concludes with a discussion on moving from an understanding of the social determinants of health to a determination to create better health, while avoiding both paternalism and fatalism—the two faces of despair that stymie effective Indigenous health policy.

Chapter 9 changes tack to consider the traditional public health protection practices based on surveillance and response. Health systems, primarily oriented to contribute to social security within the state, have an important relation to security from external threats. This includes the assurance of a healthy enough population to stock the military as well as the provision of health care to people injured by war, other organised violence and natural calamities. The chapter focuses on the health system's contribution to protection of the community from communicable diseases and its response to emergencies, then extends this analysis to consider the response to new attacks by other species and new threats to human health from the environment in which we live.

Systematic efforts to secure the safety of drinking water and the food supply go back to ancient times, and probably before. With the press of population expansion, food supply chains have become immensely long and complex. While microbiological safety remains important to prevent foodborne disease outbreaks, the energy balance and density of a community's diet must be addressed more vigorously if we are to reverse the epidemic of diet-related chronic diseases that is building in Australia and other countries. On the water front, infrastructure development has failed to keep pace with population expansion, and many communities have been caught short of water in the drought conditions that commenced around 2001 in eastern Australia. Consequently, there has been a spate of new water infrastructure projects, including recycling water for drinking and other uses. This poses a variety of very interesting challenges for public health systems and regulation.

In the event of a disaster or related emergency, health systems can respond in a number of pre-planned ways. The traditional governmentality of the emergency response draws on military models of command and control, in which available resources are commandeered from their routine operating environment and controlled through a hierarchy especially established to coordinate the response to the emergency. More recently, a new mentality has been delineated in which standard lines of control are expected to drive a surge of capacity to handle the demands arising from the emergency. Contemporary emergency response planning requires both these modes of response to be available, depending on circumstances.

REFORMING THE FUTURE

This analysis of responses to extraordinary problems can be extended to understand the response to new health problems. Examples include the epidemic of Severe Acute Respiratory Syndrome (SARS) in 2003, the looming global pandemic of novel influenza, and the obesity epidemic. Recently, planning for a global influenza pandemic has combined the traditions of communicable disease control and disaster response.

The final chapter, on health policy activism, recognises the importance of talking to consumers in the development of policy and the passion that many people have for reforming the health system. The analysis takes a view from within the health bureaucracy to examine the management of consumer consultation and the ethics of health policy activism by people working within the system.

Negotiations over health system reforms are usually hard fought by the policy and interest groups which will be affected. Adding consumers into the policy process may complicate it, but can also provide focus to the process and increase the prospect of smooth implementation. This section also considers the inherently political nature of consumer consultation and the particular management challenges this provides.

The final section considers the policy activism of people who work in public sector agencies. Working within the bureaucracy provides particular access to power, but also requires certain constraints. Insider activists are often able to set the agenda for reform debates, and frame policy so that it will actually make a positive difference. However, they must recognise the policy proclivities of the government of the day and the objectives of the organisation in which they work, both of which may be at odds with their activist orientation.

With occasional lapses, in this book I have tried not to offer concrete prescriptions for reform of the current health system. I do this constantly in my professional life, and have given enough bad policy advice to realise that the best ideas come out of an intense dialogue between a large number of well-informed and well-intentioned people, not from the private writings of individuals. If the book contributes to the enthusiasm of even a few people to engage in such debates, I will have achieved my goal.

2.

WHAT IS HEALTH?

THE NATURE OF HEALTH

The question 'What is health?' provokes debate. It doesn't help our understanding to imagine that a word has an essential meaning. Sometimes a word means one thing and sometimes another. Sometimes words are used to mean several things at once. My aim in the following discussion is not to come up with a preferred definition of health that we will use throughout the rest of this book, but to briefly characterise the sorts of definitions we find in contemporary use.

This chapter explains what we mean by health in everyday language, and in what we call the health care system. I commence with the argument that health must be acknowledged as enigmatic in some respects, as not quite definable. A second line of conceptual analysis starts from the observation that the notion of health contains its opposite: illness. Another, historical, line of analysis starts from the observation that health is understood as only desirable, that it is inconceivable that health is undesirable. The chapter concludes with a discussion showing how population health can be situated at the centre of the development of contemporary society.

Health itself has an enigmatic character. Far from being a problem, this actually facilitates the provision of health care, which includes an important dose of suggestion and occasionally a little deception both at the individual and the policy levels. These features are more important than they appear to be at first sight, and drive a number of the dynamics of the health system that we shall examine throughout the book.

There are two main strategies for constructing a definition of health. The first could be called the oppositional strategy, which takes health as the opposite of ill-health, or the absence of disease. The second could be called the displacement strategy, in which the definition is displaced to related concepts such as wellness, well-being or quality of life.

Both these definitional strategies are expressed famously in the World Health Organization definition of health: 'Health is a state of complete physical, mental and social well-being and not merely the absence of disease or infirmity' (WHO 1946, p. 1). The double negatives in the final clause—'not merely the absence of disease or infirmity'—indicate the difficulties faced by the wordsmiths of the United Nations who created the definition. Of course, the words 'disease' and 'infirmity' themselves are derived from their opposites by use of a suffix: disease and infirmity refer to the ease of living and firmness of the flesh. I shall return below to an analysis that takes off from the characteristic of the idea of health that it contains its opposite.

Palmer and Short (2000), in their excellent book on the Australian health care system, note that some people prefer to call it the 'illness care system'. They defend the term 'health care system' using the displacement strategy: 'However, if the purpose of the health care system is to undertake activities designed to promote the health status of recipients, that is, to influence the outcomes associated with health services, there is no difficulty in continuing to use this well-established terminology' (2000, p. 5).

Working with the oppositional strategy on the measurement of health and medical outcomes, Jenkinson (1994) points out that a positive, measurable definition of health can be constructed based on the measurement of either objective or subjective phenomena. Concerning objectively measurable things, he comments: 'The biomedical model of ill health is rooted in a belief that ill health is an objective, measurable state. This is a disease-based view of ill health, in which poor health is a function of an abnormality' (1994, p. 1). He contrasts this with a definition of illness based on subjective, but still measurable, states: 'Illness, on the other hand, refers to a person's subjective experience of "ill health" and is indicated by reported symptoms and subjective accounts in terms of pain, distress, discomfort, and the like' (1994, p. 1).

The objective and the subjective definitions cannot be considered to be mutually exclusive. As Jenkinson notes: 'It is, for example, possible to feel ill without any signs of an underlying disease, and possible to have disease without any subjective awareness of illness' (1994, p. 2). He also notes that this point is easily understood by the general public, and accords with the findings of Herzlich's (1973) study on lay concepts of health and disease that, among lay people, 'health was regarded as something multidimensional: the absence of disease, a positive state of wellbeing, and a "reserve" of overall health, determined in large part by individual constitution' (1973, quoted in Jenkinson 1994, p. 3). On this view, people could define themselves as healthy while knowing they had a serious illness, even while they were suffering with it. It is in this way that people with serious disabilities or chronic infections such as HIV can talk about 'keeping themselves healthy'.

It is easy to see health as something valuable. Much health policy argument is based on the premise that health is characterised as only desirable, that health cannot be undesirable. The fact that such argument at least appears plausible makes us realise that it has become unusual these days to define health in the value-free terms once preferred by philosophers of natural science. In the 1970s, Boorse summarised the case for the previously mainstream argument that 'health as absence of disease is a value-free theoretical notion. Its main elements are biological function and statistical normality . . . This conception of health is as value free as biological function' (Boorse 1977, p. 542). This is an important tradition that continues to underpin vast amounts of research activity. For example, epidemiological studies typically seek to understand the way events have an effect on health, but health itself is rarely defined as an outcome in these studies. Usually, specific phenomena are taken as the outcomes of interest (e.g. death, or myocardial infarction, or a respondent's answer to a question about how they feel). From the standpoint of epidemiological practice, 'health' can be considered merely a class name for the collection of outcome phenomena the epidemiologist investigates (see Miettinen 1985, Ch. 2).

While there are many advantages arising from the nineteenth century positivist tradition of attempting to be value free in scientific investigations—not least because an injection of scientists' values rarely makes anyone feel better—it is not possible to extend this tradition to a broader understanding of health. Gadamer (1996) has explained why in an interesting way: 'It strikes me as extremely significant that in today's highly developed technical civilization it has proved necessary to invent an expression like the "quality of life" . . . this expression reflects a fundamental and immemorial human recognition that each of us has to "lead" our own lives, that we must decide for ourselves how we are going to live' (1996, p. 104). Gadamer points out that sickness and health are important precisely because they are bound up with this matter of how people lead their lives, an inherently normative, moral and ethical matter that cannot be conceived as value free.

People providing health care do so in a complex ethical environment. There are two meanings of the word 'treat' in this context, as Duckett (2004) has noted: 'Complaints lodged against doctors are often about the way in which the patient was treated, not in the medical sense of the word but in terms of the respect shown by the doctor to the patient' (2004, pp. xxii–xxiii). Gadamer comments that: 'Treatment always involves a certain granting of freedom. It does not just consist in laying down regulations or writing out prescriptions. For the doctor it is fairly clear what it means to say that someone is undergoing treatment with them. It involves a certain responsibility but at the same time a certain care which must recognize the freedom of the patient' (1996, p. 104).

Health, rather than being definable in some complex way, is fundamentally enigmatic: there is something about it that always sits beyond clear conceptual grasp. In part, the enigmatic character of health may be because health is something to be desired, and this desirability is bound up with an inability to know it completely. We desire health both for its own sake, and because when we have it our ability to do things and to enjoy living is enhanced. It enhances our capacity to desire other things. The desire for health is one-sided: we feel that to desire less health would be irrational, perhaps even unhealthy. The desire for health is social because we seek health from others, through their services, prescriptions and other advice. We also desire health for others, feel that they should desire it and pursue it for themselves, and will release them from other social obligations to do so.

Most of us can say when we feel healthy: when we sense no immediate problems with our physical embodiment and feel able to do things and enjoy doing them. So the concept of health expresses, on the one hand, a lack (of bodily problems) and, on the other, a capacity (to do and enjoy things). But these are the negative and the positive corollaries of health, not health itself.

The enigmatic character of health is at the heart of health care. Health care of course shares this characteristic with religion and magic. Rivers (1924), a physician and an influential anthropologist of medicine in the early twentieth century, has offered a definition of each that shows their similarity and difference. In a series of lectures to the Royal College of Physicians in

London, he noted that each implies a mechanism of efficacy, and that the different mechanism of efficacy between religion, magic and medicine is in fact the major point of divergence between the practices in the three fields.

Rivers defined religion as 'a group of processes, the efficacy of which depends on the will of some higher power, the power of whose intervention is sought by rites of supplication and propitiation' (1924, p. 4). Magic, on the other hand, can be defined as 'a group of processes in which man uses rites which depend for their efficacy on his own power, or on powers believed to be inherent in, or the attributes of, certain objects and processes which are used in these rites' (1924, p. 4). Both religion and magic, then, are technologies for making the world more favourable for the practitioner or their client; religion is a technology that motivates a transcendental power, and magic is a technology that mobilises powers immanent in the practitioner or other worldly things woven into the magic.

Medicine, like magic and unlike religion, deals with this-worldly things. Like magic, it consists of practices designed to produce a beneficial effect through an understanding of humans as part of nature. It is directed to control a specific group of phenomena 'viz. those especially affecting man himself, which so influence his behaviour as to unfit him for the normal accomplishment of his physical and social functions—phenomena which lower his vitality and tend towards death' (Rivers 1924, p. 4). The practice of medicine is about avoiding or treating disease and injury, and the measure of its success is the health of the patient. Rivers goes on to give a key insight into the definition of disease: 'By a process of generalization, society has come to classify these phenomena together, and has distinguished them from other groups of natural phenomena under the name of disease' (1924, p. 4).

While the logical relations given by Rivers are theoretical and can be applied to all societies, he supposes that in primitive societies there is less systematic distinction between the three. The concept of disease may not be restricted to natural causes. Through anthropological study of indigenous peoples in Melanesia, New Guinea and Australia, Rivers showed how religious and magical thinking was actually rational if we recognise that the beliefs of the thinkers form the premises of this rationality. He also showed how specific practices diffused between cultures, sometimes taking on a religious character, and sometimes a medical character. For example, he suggests that bloodletting, which was introduced into the Pacific islands from west to east, has a largely therapeutic character in Melanesia, but in

Polynesia—a highly religious culture—it has been taken up into religious ceremony and social custom, while continuing to be used in some ways for therapeutic purposes (Rivers 1924, p. 91).

In our own culture, disease is an important phenomenon towards which religious and superstitious practices are directed. Some religious practices, such as ritual hand-washing, have also (thankfully) found their way into medical practice. The logic of medical thinking also includes religious and magical elements. This can clearly be seen in the formulation of prognosis. The physician can rely on empirical studies and probability thinking to define the risk of relapse in a patient with cancer. But when the patient says, 'Doctor, I understand the probabilities, but will *I* relapse?', the physician usually concedes that the answer is in the lap of the gods.

A principal factor relating the efficacy of medical, magical and religious interventions is the place of suggestion within all three technologies. The efficacy of suggestion is rooted in the shared values and understandings of a culture, which underpin the believability of the suggestions and the authority of the person making the suggestion. More problematically, as Rivers points out, 'with this real factor of suggestion there is mixed up much deception, especially on the part of those to whose special knowledge the production and cure of disease is ascribed' (1924, p. 47). An important part of the art of medicine is in turning the patient's desire for health into a striving for life itself. Knowingly misleading patients is part of the stock in trade of doctors, both in the use of suggestion and in not unduly worrying patients by informing them of unpleasant future developments. These deceptions affect patients' propensity to strive for health and no doubt often make a contribution to the course of an illness turning out well, especially in the hands of a highly skilled doctor. Of course, if things turn out badly and the deception is unmasked, the doctor could be in hot water, but most skilled (and, I would argue, ethical) doctors see this at times as a risk worth taking in the interests of maximising the chances of benefit to the patient. By its nature, this aspect of medical practice is not amenable to rigorous empirical study or codification of practice.

The provision of health care is thus complicated by the enigmatic character of health, the way health underpins the conduct of our lives, the anxiety the possibility of losing health provokes in many people, the complexity of medical science, and the often quite incomplete level of knowledge on both sides of the therapeutic relationship between patients and their doctors.

In passing, I would like to note some of the implications for financial transactions surrounding health care. This topic is treated in more detail in Chapter 3. The enigmatic character of health and the therapeutic importance of suggestion by experts combine with the complexity of health knowledge to produce a profound information asymmetry surrounding transactions between doctors and patients, and has over time produced a quite peculiar set of arrangements for the financial side of those transactions. Health is highly desirable but cannot itself be contracted for. At the individual level, we receive health services and advice with the recognition that these may or may not improve our health, and that even if they do we may not be able to tell. At the societal level it is much the same, with attempts to contract organisations to deliver better health outcomes largely having been unsuccessful: because population health outcomes are difficult to attribute to particular interventions, health outcome measures do not work very well for giving accounts of organisational performance.

Recognition that health is enigmatic can help our analysis of the different perspectives that health professionals, their patients and the patients' carers all bring to specific episodes of health care provision, advice-giving or personal action for health. It also helps explain the endless innovation in health technology, systems of care and personal motivations directed towards being healthy or becoming healthier. This will be a recurring issue throughout the book.

HEALTH DISCIPLINES

Turning from a conceptual to an historical lens, health can be understood as the notion underpinning the development of the various health disciplines and systems in modernity. Each of the disciplines of health (surgery, nursing, physiotherapy, public health, and so on) has sought to create a field of science coupled with a field of practice directed towards the betterment of Man. A glance at the spirit of enlightenment in the early 1800s helps us understand this historical expression of the notion of progress through knowledge as a grand humanistic project.

In nineteenth century thinking, the notion of health provides a motive force for the development of social activities, the main moments of which can be summarised as: the attainment of knowledge about health; the application of this knowledge through judgments about health in specific cases; resulting in the determination of practices that promote health.

Nineteenth and twentieth century developments in health have produced a vast proliferation of health sciences intent on the attainment of knowledge, health professions concerned with the development of a capacity for making judgments about health, and a series of health-related institutions through which health professionals practise. These knowledges, professions and institutions display various humanist orientations: they take 'Man' as their subject; they are committed to generating progress through the scientific discovery and application of knowledge; and they have been incorporated into various humanist programs of government— for example by the Fabians in the United Kingdom and Australia.

The question 'What is health?' is often posed in the expectation that the answer will capture some fundamental essence of the human condition. Here we are exploring another sort of answer—a recent history of the idea of health. This different kind of answer strives to reveal why health has become one of the most prevalent metaphors in modernity, and shows how the term is often used to render various social objectives unproblematic. This can help uncover the hidden operation of power within the knowledge discourses of the health sciences and health professions, because it alerts us to the analytical problem that we may have been deceived by power—that that is what power does.

A traditional question, 'What is health?' traditionally elicits a number of different types of answers. To briefly summarise:

- The World Health Organization offers a self-contained, all-encompassing definition: health is 'a state of complete physical, mental and social well-being, and not merely the absence of disease or infirmity' (WHO 1946).
- Health economics texts debate whether health is an end in itself, or a state of being that enables the person to pursue other ends.
- Physicians make their definition in the negative: health *is* the absence of disease or infirmity. In this sense, the measures of health are the inverse of measures of morbidity and mortality (for a sympathetic treatment of this position, see Boorse 1977).
- More recently, the psychometricians have developed methods for the subjective estimation of feelings or judgments of healthiness along a number of quality of life dimensions (Jenkinson 1994).

Whatever their differences, these definitions of health share a certain earnestness. Another set of definitions attempt to define 'health' as the beginning of a critique:

- It is frequently observed that the health system concerns itself with illness.
- The critique of the health professions traditionally begins by noting their concern for the pathological.

These definitions share a sense of irony as a propulsive force for the development of the critique. However, the irony in these critiques is quickly overtaken by another earnestness in their concern for a better approach to social progress. This may be unavoidable, of course, and this book is probably no exception. More interesting is that both types of definition point to a common characteristic of the concept of health: it contains a definition of its opposite, of illness or the unhealthy. This characteristic raises the possibility that the question 'What is health?' can be answered in a speculative spirit, in which enlightening ideas propel history by coordinating the actions of their adherents. In the enlightenment world view of the early nineteenth century, mental and physical things were understood as different manifestations of the same substance. Things—physical and mental—have an immediacy about them, and this immediacy is their being. Their being reflects their essence or, to put it the other way around, the essence of things reflects their being: being is intelligible because its essence is understandable. In simplistic terms, through the dialectical logic of thesis, antithesis and synthesis, being is the thesis, essence the antithesis, and the notion the synthesis of being and essence. Being is the immediate, and essence is the reflection of being. Readers who studied a little of the German philosopher Hegel (1770–1831) will recognise this style of reasoning.

Let's look at the similarities with the question 'What is truth?' This was Pilate's old and hopeless question to his deicidal subjects (John 18:38). We could note that the condition of possibility for Pilate's question was twofold: first, he held the supreme governing power in the place where he framed the question; and second, the matter he was arbitrating concerned whether Jesus was a higher power. Truth was the defining obsession of the enlightenment. From its advances in science, its philosophy, the realist turn of art and the decline of superstition and religion, 'What is truth?' has been the heuristic question underpinning many philosophical systems. It is a peculiar kind of question. It has many similarities—grammar at least—with the question 'What is health?' In the history of philosophy, philosophers prior to the nineteenth century idealists 'might well have agreed that no more need be said than the *Shorter Oxford English Dictionary's* definition of "truth": "conformity with the facts, agreement with reality"' (Flew 1979, p. 329). Since then, thinking about truth has become more complicated as it has assumed a foundational role within philosophy. From a moral perspective, it has been difficult to see truth as undesirable. This has been done, of course, by a number of courageous thinkers: the playwright Ibsen showed its undesirability in the tightly wound family structures of nineteenth century society (e.g. Ibsen 1981); Nietzsche (1966) showed its bloody and violent origins; and Foucault (e.g. 1997) showed how a quest for truth could be used to deceive. Such thinkers, however, were readily branded as antisocial and somewhat dangerous misfits. Their critics exhibit a morally driven mindset from a world where truths are told most honestly in the confession.

The Enlightenment philosophers asked the question 'What is truth?' in their concern to understand the essence of being. The nineteenth century humanists asked 'What is health?' in their concern with the essence of humanity—referred to as 'Man'. The object of humanist interest, reflection, thought and practice is Man. In particular, for nineteenth century humanism, the immediate object of interest is Man in his species being. The essence of Man is his life: the reflection of his being in living; a living and a life that is qualitatively different from that of all other species. For the enlightened nineteenth century humanist, this living is historically embedded: living is the reflective practice of becoming. It is in this light that we can say that the truth of Man is health. For what is health? According to the World Health Organization, it is 'a state of complete physical, mental and social well-being' (WHO 1946). Health is the essence of being a complete person, able to live a complete life. Health is the most fundamental condition of freedom. Freedom is the mode through which one's health is related to other aspects of life: health bestows freedom of movement without disability, freedom of social engagement without handicap, and freedom of enjoyment without pain. Under the notion of health, living beings presuppose their capacity for life, and actively live their life in relation to others. Health is life presupposing its powers in its acts of living in the world; health gives human beings the power and activity to live in the world.

I have laboured with this elaboration of the notion of health, showing how it emerges from the ground of humanity's being and essence, to point out some of the relations between this style of thought and the development of health-related knowledges and practices from the nineteenth century on.

Enlightenment knowledge develops through the elaboration of subjective judgments and syllogistic forms. It achieves objectivity in the comprehension of nature in its mechanical structure, chemical or genetic principles, and natural purposes. The nineteenth century concept of life had an especially human sense: a concern for life as principle, as soul or spirit; the life left out by 'man as machine' metaphors generated in eighteenth century enlightenment thinking. As the nineteenth century progressed, there was an increasing recognition of the embodiment of human life, concerned with embodied humans as labouring beings.

In a fundamental sense, each of the health sciences and health professions emanates from an idea about health. Consider the following examples. The idea of medicine that developed towards the end of the nineteenth century was the therapeutic possibilities based on understanding the intersection of the germ principle of disease with the genetic principle of life (see Chapter 4). The idea of physiotherapy is to know the therapeutic effect of external manipulations of the body, and to apply this knowledge in the practice of physiotherapy. The idea of occupational therapy is to understand and act on the therapeutic possibilities that arise because life is work. The contemporary idea of public health is to elucidate and propagate social arrangements conducive to the health of the species. This can be seen in the definition of public health offered by the Public Health Association of Australia: 'Public Health is a combination of science, practical skills, and beliefs that is directed to the maintenance and improvement of the health of all people. It is one of the efforts organised by society to protect, promote, and restore the people's health through collective or social actions' (Public Health Association of Australia 1997, p. 2).

Each idea of health is elaborated as a new knowledge and a new practice, contributing to the perfection of the species being. This is done as a concrete activity in the laborious development over time of the knowledges and practices of the health professions. These health sciences and health disciplines are directed in a humanist program towards increasing the freedom of people to live life as they please.

POPULATION HEALTH AND POLITICS

While this Enlightenment perspective is still a common and powerful motivator of scientific, practical and policy endeavour in the health field, it is also helpful to come to grips with a broader analysis that gets outside of our desire to help or make progress and goes beyond the health field to show how population health can be situated at the centre of a broader social analysis.

Thinking back to the definitions of health discussed in the last section, they all share a striking absence or lack: health is not considered as problematic in itself. The problems relating to health in the above definitions can only be posed in relation to the means of attaining better health, or the problems associated with the absence of health. Health itself always appears as something unproblematically desirable. Everybody wants health, for who could want less health? Even health-reducing activities—such as smoking cigarettes or water pollution—are strangled within the health discourse without a whisper: health-reducing activities, far from rendering health problematic, are themselves rendered pathological. For example, the habit of smoking tobacco is rendered as an addiction at the same moment it is recognised as bad for health.

Just as the curiosity that the notion of health contains its opposite pointed to the value of a dialectical analysis, so this lack of undesirability in the concept of health draws our attention to another analytical strategy: the history of how that idea came to be so unquestionable. We can call this sort of history of an idea a genealogy.

Genealogies are useful for problematising seemingly unproblematic concepts and seemingly unchallengeable ideas by tracing the historical events in the discursive formation of such concepts. They show the historical power struggles which resulted in the formation of the concept under scrutiny in its field of knowledge, and enable a strategic reading of the concept within contemporary discourse to lay bare the often highly problematic power struggles in which the concept is deployed.

Foucault was deeply interested in the development of systems of thought, in particular with the systems of thought prevalent in the fields of health and security during the nineteenth century that so shaped the institutional forms of contemporary western society. Foucault has, following Nietzsche, contributed to the genealogy of humanism and enlightenment. His progress on this topic in *The Order of Things* (Foucault

1990a) established his academic notoriety. It was in this work that he raised the prospect of the end of Man, meaning the end of the humanist programs based on the socially constructed object of 'Man', following his exposé of 'Man' as merely (?!) a foundational concept of modernity (Foucault 1990a, p. 370). In a later text he cautions against any simple interpretation of humanism, noting that the word has identified many movements at many different times, with many and often conflicting characteristics (Foucault 1997, p. 314).

In this analysis, I have been most interested in the humanism that emerged in the mid-nineteenth century. This particular humanism was an heir to the Enlightenment: it propagated a dream of the perfectibility of humanity through science. Despite Foucault's warning, I think this is the humanism in which he too was most interested.

In ancient times, the patriarch of the household had the power of life and death over the members of the household, although it could only legitimately be exercised if there was a threat to the life or way of life of the patriarch or their sovereign: if the law had been broken, death could be the punishment; or if external enemies threatened, subjects could be sent to war, thus exposing their lives. 'The right which was formulated [in Roman law] as the "power of life and death" was in reality the right to *take* life or *let* live. Its symbol, after all, was the sword' (Foucault 1976, p. 136).

Around the time from the Enlightenment to the birth of the Industrial Revolution, the sovereign's power over life and death changed from a solely subtractive power—where life could be taken or not taken—to a power that could also be deployed positively. It was now a power that could 'incite, reinforce, control, monitor, optimize, and organize' (Foucault 1976, p. 136). This is not so much power by might, or even power by right (as the sovereign and their court would like it seen), but power by knowledge, by know-how.

The use of death also became intensified, with war becoming not so much a violent engagement between sovereigns as a contest between populations, with genocides and holocausts emerging as stock tactics. 'Wars are no longer waged in the name of a sovereign who must be defended; they are waged on behalf of the existence of everyone; entire populations are mobilized for the purpose of wholesale slaughter in the name of life necessity: massacres have become vital' (Foucault 1976, p. 137). The techniques of surgery and of population health owe much to the theatres of war, and have on occasion contributed a technological edge to one side or other.

This emergence of population as a field for the play of social power, both in war and in generative pursuits, was associated with the rise of a democratic approach to the definition of a people, and accompanied a shift from monarchic to democratic forms of state: 'the existence in question is no longer the juridical existence of sovereignty; at stake is the biological existence of a population' (Foucault 1976, p. 137).

Foucault coined the term 'biopower' for this assemblage of social power exercised over populations of people which emerged in the modern period. This is a useful concept in the understanding of the development of western states. It helps explain the remarkable fact that the institutions of health care are among the largest of the modern state: the health portfolio in Australian state governments accounts for around one-third of total state financial outlays. It helps explain the political prominence of problems such as birth rate, longevity, housing and migration. It helps explain the drive and innovation exhibited in the development of the techniques of population control, including health care provision, through the development of the disciplines of medicine, nursing care, physical therapies, sanitation, genetics (and eugenics), health promotion and emergency management. These and other technologies of population became central to the development of the modern state, the development of the sciences and practices of modern health care.

The humanist program for the development of health sciences and practices was built on a transcendental ethics based on universal principles, a transcendental practice based on scientific knowledge and transcendental knowledge based on scientific practice. This transcendentalism is rooted in a conception of the human spirit and human history that in practice continually fails the implementers of the humanist project it underpins, a humanist project infected by the Enlightenment attempts to use science and disciplines to pursue the social conditions of progress. However, successful medicine through science has come often enough that the project has maintained its momentum. Governments still appeal for electoral legitimacy by promising to bring the latest technological breakthroughs to the public system. Progress or the promise of progress remains high on the best buy lists in the competition for policy attention and remains a great motivator of the research/policy nexus, which we will explore in the next chapter.

In summary, this chapter has explored the nature of health and the role the idea of health plays in state and society. I have argued, following

Gadamer, that human health is fundamentally enigmatic, and that this gives the concrete activities related to health a flexibility and creativity that has enabled a close and evolving relationship between health practices and the living of life itself. I have tried to show how the idea of 'health' as a humanist notion has underpinned the development in modernity of the multitude of health disciplines that combine scientific inquiry with professional practice in a strategy of human progress. Finally, we examined Foucault's claims for the field of biopower, that the health of populations has been a central concern of the state in modern society. From this perspective, the health-related activities of government, or health stewardship, can be understood as not just one of an ever-growing list of areas of government activity, but a core responsibility bound up with the viability of contemporary society itself.

3.

HEALTH POLICY

It is one thing to argue why the state should take an interest in health and make health policy. It is another to understand how public policy is made and how it shapes things in society.

Modern western democracies regard the health of their citizens as crucial to the continuance of the state itself. In the last chapter, I introduced this idea with Foucault's term of 'biopower', describing an assemblage of powers and technologies orientated to keeping the population in good health.

The importance of health to democracy cannot be overrated, as evidenced by the fact that the institutions of health care are among the largest of the modern state. This is well illustrated in Australia by the observation that the health portfolio in Australian state governments accounts for around one-third of total state financial outlays.

Any understanding of health and policy matters has to recognise that health care is fundamentally related to the powers and responsibilities of the elected component of government. State power underpins our health policies, which have the objective of ensuring the health of citizens is looked after. This democratic objective is the basis for the health stewardship role of governments.

This chapter discusses general issues of public policy and health. It begins by considering the powers of the state and the operationalisation of state power through public policy and public financing. It then examines the relationship between policy and research, and the changing relations between medical knowledge, health insurance and public finance in the assemblage of the health system. It concludes by considering the neo-liberal approach to the regulation of freedom in health system reform, with reference to the introduction of Australia's Medicare policy in 1983/84.

GOVERNMENTALITY IN THE LIBERAL STATE

The activities of health departments in most western democracies are fundamentally related to the powers and responsibilities of the elected component of government—in Australia's case, the cabinet, including the health minister. Duly selected cabinet ministers are given executive commissions by the head of state—the state governors and the Governor-General—to operate the machinery of state. Health departments are that part of the machinery that provides advice about policy to the ministers and cabinet of the day, and that executes government policy directives.

The neologism 'governmentality' was invented by Foucault in an introductory lecture to his seminar series of 1978 at the College de France entitled 'Security, Territory and Population' (Foucault 1991, see esp. p. 102; Gordon 1991). Because Foucault did so much work in the history of medicine and health systems, it is perhaps not surprising that his headline governmental themes of security, territory and population are central to understanding the dynamics of governing the modern health system and the health of populations. The desire for security in the face of uncertainty about one's health drove the development of the health insurance system and the increasing role of the state in financing health services. The delineation of geographical territory is central to the traditional public health techniques of responding to epidemics and of quarantine; of what we might call the village doctor ideal of general practice; and of the modern administration of the health system through area health services. Finally, the governmental focus on populations relies to a large extent on the population sciences, the major developments in which have occurred within the family of public health disciplines.

Since the age of revolutions in Europe, government has been conceived as contiguous with the forms of social control and discipline that regulate culture and social structure within society. No longer is rule conducted by a sovereign who imposes his will on the people: the King's head has been cut off and modern government is of the people, by the people and for the people, and occurs through a wide variety of techniques. This is obviously extremely problematic in practice.

In contrast to the more traditional focus of political theory on moral theories of sovereignty and legitimacy in the democratic state, the focus for recent analyses of government has been the problems of governmental administration, its fields of application, its purposes and its techniques as they are determined by the structure of society and as they in turn shape that society. At its best, this style of analysis recasts administrative science as the central discipline of political theory, expanding its ambit to address the main themes of politics so that studies of administration and public policy are understood as theories of governing rather than as subsidiary disciplines to theories of sovereignty.

Traditional accounts of government contrast the ideology of liberalism, including the high value it places on individual freedom, with the practical operation of governments to limit this freedom. The style of account I have adopted is no less concerned with the issue of freedom, but analyses the principle of maximum freedom not as the central plank of a liberal ideology but as an objective in the administrative technologies of government, as an idea that in a practical way guides a particular mode of governing. Barry Hindess, my politics teacher at the Australian National University, described this analytical shift as follows:

> Liberalism is commonly understood as a political doctrine or ideology concerned with the maximization of individual liberty and, in particular, with the defence of that liberty against the state. However, following Foucault's work on governmentality, a different usage has been suggested, based on the idea of a liberal mode of government. This usage suggests first that the sphere of individual liberty should be seen, not so much as reflecting the natural liberty of the individual, but rather as a governmental product (Hindess 1996, pp. 300–1).

The agencies of the state in liberal societies are themselves primarily concerned with conducting the conduct of government in other fields: 'Liberal government identifies a domain outside "politics", and seeks to manage it without destroying its existence and its autonomy. This is made possible through the activities and calculations of a proliferation of independent agents including philanthropists, doctors, hygienists, managers, planners, parents, and social workers' (Rose and Miller 1992, p. 180).

With the shift of state power from the sovereign to the people, and the rise of democratic forms of social organisation, the health of the population shifted from being a resource for the city-state in the pursuit of extra-territorial policy objectives to being something that the state attempted to govern through domestic policy. Certainly, a healthy population continued to be an important resource for the waging of war, and grew in importance as a source of labour from the Industrial Revolution on. Even today, labour-oriented migration programs ensure that those allowed to immigrate are healthy so that the health of migrants in Australia is significantly better than the health of those born in Australia. But the health objectives of the modern state are now more oriented to ensuring that the health of citizens is looked after.

THE AUSTRALIAN STATE AND THE GOVERNMENT OF HEALTH

The idea of the state has been elaborated in political theory, and is different from but overlaps with the idea of the public sector discussed in economic theory. Glyn Davis, a distinguished Australian political theorist and policy practitioner, has defined the state as 'an ensemble of agencies of legitimate coercion and as an amalgamated set of collective resources which intentionally and unintentionally produce policy outcomes' (Davis et al. 1993, p. 18). The agencies of coercion include the armed forces, the police and the prisons. At the end of the day, the state can and does physically force its citizens to comply with its policies. One example from the history of the health system occurred in the days before the introduction of Medicare in the early 1970s. Bankruptcy laws were such that non-payment of debts could result in imprisonment, and this was regularly enforced. What is most interesting is that in 1972 the most common cause of imprisonment for unpaid debts was for unpaid health care debts!

The network of state coercion does not usually need to physically coerce people to comply with health policy—the fact that it can is usually enough. Nevertheless, when making policy it is important to keep in mind that in the case of policies where implementation is underpinned by the possibility of state-sponsored physical violence, the government must truly be convinced that the merits of the policy warrant such force. Empirically, it seems clear that such policies can produce better health system operation (Braithwaite and Drahos 2000; Braithwaite, Makkai and Braithwaite 2007).

No state is a unitary structure. The Australian state has three formal levels of government: Commonwealth, state and local. Davis et al. (1993)

have accurately described it as 'an entwined federation based on regional power at the state level with a prescribed set of powers transferred to the Commonwealth level' (1993, p. 23). The state includes a large number of institutions, including parliaments, governments (each comprised of a cabinet and various ministries), courts, armed forces, departments (including health departments), services (such as hospitals and schools), the Reserve Bank, the Tax Office, statutory authorities (such as the universities and the Australian Institute of Health and Welfare) and government-owned business enterprises (such as Medibank Private at the time of writing). Public hospitals may be a part of a Department of Health (as in New South Wales and the Australian Capital Territory) or a separate service with their own board of management established by the government—sometimes by administrative direction and sometimes by statute.

Public policy has been defined in many ways, all of which include the idea that public policy is made by governments and affects members of the public (people or corporations). Governments can make decisions (e.g. cabinet decisions or ministers' decisions) and can act (e.g. ministers may introduce legislation into the parliament or give an order to a department or statutory authority). Members of the government and political commentators tend to refer to announced government decisions as policies, while bureaucrats and policy analysts tend to interpret the actions (and inactions) of governments as policy. When governments act on their decisions, the two interpretations coincide. However, when departments act on the basis of previous governments' actions (e.g. legislation), or when governments do not act on announced decisions or act on decisions that have not been announced, the two types of interpretations can contradict one another. In this book, the particular meaning I am giving to the word 'policy' will be clear from the context. In general, I use the terms 'policy' or 'public policy' to mean the rules for action, in place at a particular time for the institutions of state, that have arisen from the actions of governments present and past.

The executive government of Australia comprises the Governor-General in executive council and the departments of state established by the parliament. The executive council is made of ministers drawn from the parliament appointed by the Governor-General on the advice of a prime minister who commands a majority of members on the floor of the House of Representatives (Australian Constitution, Chapters 1 and 2). The ministers administer, but are not part of, their departments.

The Australian Constitution defines departments as a part of the executive government. Nevertheless, there is a clear divide between the elected ministers and the unelected appointed public servants who have only the authority delegated to them by the parliament. While (senior) public servants can themselves make policy, they do so within the authority allowed them by the minister, cabinet and parliament. The rein can be fairly loose—for example, in the internal operation of hospitals or the use of statutory powers by public health officials. However, over the last 30 years there has been a tightening of the policy grip by elected officials, coupled with a more hands-off approach to managerial or operational matters.

In the field of health, the state cannot directly provide health to the public. It can provide services and other things that may improve the public's health, but it cannot provide health itself. This is different to the situation in many other fields, where the state can, if it chooses, provide education, extract tax, provide pensions, allow or stop immigration, and so on. Because of this special feature of the government of health, it makes sense to talk of the object of health policy in general terms as health stewardship. This is a bit like the stewards at a horse race. They marshal the horses, set the starting barrier, photograph the finish and judge the winner. They do not race, and most do not even ride, but without them it would be Rafferty's rules, with little chance of a fair bet and no chance of a horse racing industry.

Health departments are intimately involved with the policy process, and have much influence because of this. Much senior executive time is spent designing the channels for the creation, transmission to the government, approval and return of policy papers. They can ask their minister to make policy according to their advice. Consequently, much of the actual work of policy units in health departments consists of preparing advice for and receiving direction back from the health minister. Even cabinet submissions are prepared for the minister, because it is the minister who takes material to cabinet, not the department.

Once a government has made policy, it falls to departments to administer it. There is considerable scope in such administration to influence things, as many government policies contain considerable scope for interpretation during implementation (departments, of course, may have provided advice to the effect that the department should be given considerable scope for interpretation of the policy). This can give scope for tactics and responsiveness during implementation—for example, to achieve meshing in with existing policy. On the definition of public policy given above, the departments set much of the detail of the rules for action.

STRUCTURE AND REGULATION

Taking a somewhat simplistic view, the fields of policy action include the structure of health systems and services; the regulation of health care activities; and health care financing by state treasuries and other means. Of course these three fields interact—for example, in the heavy regulation of private spending on health care. However, each of these three fields has its own history and logic, and these need to be understood as determining the possibilities for policy in any particular debate where reform is being considered.

Loosely, policy concerning structure relates to the management of the health system, and regulation is historically a key tool for the policy influence over the expertise of health professionals and private sector financing in the health system. After discussing these matters, along with a consideration of the relationship between research and policy, the final section of this chapter puts together the overall assemblage of the health system from the components of management, expertise and financing.

The structure of the Australian health system is complex, comprising interwoven components operated by the Commonwealth, the states, non-government organisations and private sector companies and individuals. There are a number of excellent overviews of the structure of Australia's health system (AIHW 2006; Duckett 2004; Palmer and Short 2000), and many specific aspects of this structure will be discussed in the following chapters. Briefly, the Commonwealth's pharmaceutical and medical benefits schemes underpin much of the structure of private professional health care businesses while the states license health professionals and operate most of the free public hospitals, with religious organisations operating the rest and private companies owning the pay-as-you-go hospitals. Mutual corporations provide health insurance. Global pharmaceutical, medical device, and information technology companies are the main providers of specialised health care products. There is also a large buy-in to health care from other domestic industries providing buildings, transport, linen, cleaning, communications, education, and so on.

State governments structure health services in the public sector through direct ownership and management, and influence the structure of private sector services through regulation and financing arrangements. The structure of state government-provided services is a major outcome and preoccupation of state government policy. The current dominant mode of organisation for state government services is geographical area-based management of all health services provided by the government in that region. The exact delineation of which state government services are administered within health areas and which are provided through other portfolios (e.g. community services) varies from time to time and from state to state. The split of health-related services between state government and local government is more stable, with local government generally providing environmental health services and regulation of food businesses, assurance of health-promoting design features within town and regional planning, and some health-related community development (e.g. provision of support for self-help groups).

Even within a single jurisdiction, there are many possibilities for structuring publicly provided health services. Services can be managed as divisions within health departments. This is efficient in small jurisdictions but can become unwieldy in large states (although technically it has become the case in New South Wales, with the restructure of 2005), where the 'department' can employ over 100 000 people. An argument against such an internal arrangement is that the mode of operation of the department in its mission to serve the government of the day may not be the optimal mode of operation for its additional mission of providing health services.

To avoid such a compromise, many health services are established by statute as separate organisations. The form of these statutory health service organisations could be managed by a statutory chief executive, or by a board appointed by the government or perhaps elected from the local community under rules specified in the statute. The statute may require accountability to the department, to the minister or to the parliament, or may not specify it at all.

The history of health administration in Australian states has been marked by repeated swings in the governance of health services between a departmental operations approach and the independent statutory authority approach, with various levels of managerial autonomy in between. These policy swings are influenced by the politics of account-ability (e.g. consider whose problem it is perceived to be to manage waiting lists), the possibility of cost savings, ideology, administrative fashion and the need for change in a stagnant organisation.

Another structure common at the Commonwealth level of government is the benefit scheme, where a benefit is provided to an individual. The Medicare benefits scheme pays a cash reimbursement to a patient for a service on the Medicare benefits schedule provided by a doctor, optometrist, nurse, psychologist, physiotherapist, occupational therapist or diabetes educator. The Pharmaceutical Benefits Scheme provides patients with medications prescribed by a medical practitioner. Interestingly, the benefit is not cash but the medication itself. The Commonwealth reimburses the dispensing pharmacist for the retail cost of the drug (and pays a dispensing fee).

Benefits schemes allow patients to choose their own provider, and so facilitate the development of a market for the services or products for which there is a benefit. The government retains detailed control over access to this market by both producers and consumers, and detailed control over prices and other aspects of the transactions. Such a structure provides many avenues for policy intervention, including to set up the conditions for market transactions to aggregate into the distributional efficiencies which policy-makers seek from market arrangements.

Patterns of regulation in the health system are best observed in a longer timeframe than structural patterns. The current regulation of health professionals in Australia continues a style of government that was established in the states prior to Federation. Pensabene (1980) and Willis (1983) have documented this in Victoria, Lloyd (1994) for New South Wales, and White (1999) for South Australia. Essentially, the medical profession in Australia was founded on a set of regulations that provide registration for medical practitioners, and prohibit those who are not registered from claiming that they are medical practitioners. Registration is largely controlled by the profession itself in three ways: control over training in medical schools, with a medical degree being required for provisional registration; control over hospital practice, with at least one year of acceptable supervised practice in a hospital being required for full registration; and control by medical practitioners over the proceedings of the registration boards themselves, including the exercise of their disciplinary and exclusionary powers. Since the 1960s, this regime has been extended to provide for specialist training through supervised practice after initial registration; by the turn of the millennium, a non-specialist career in medicine had become a thing of the past (see the discussion on medical licensing in Chapter 4).

There have been two major sociological interpretations of this mode of governing medical practice. The American sociologist Talcott Parsons argued in the 1950s that it was part of fostering an ethos of professionalism amongst medical practitioners whereby they shouldered their responsibility to do their best for their patients—including training and disciplining their own—and in return they (and their patients) were protected from the raw competition of untrained practitioners. The patient:

> is not only generally not in a position to do what needs to be done, but he does not 'know' what needs to be done or how to do it. It is not merely that he, being bedridden, cannot go down to the drug store to get what is needed, but that he would, even if well, not be qualified to do what is needed, and to judge what needs to be done . . . And one of the most serious disabilities of the layman is that he is not qualified to judge technical qualifications in general or in detail (Parsons 1952, p. 441).

This line was restated by the British social theorist Thomas Osborne (1993) in the 1990s as a classical example of the liberal mode of government, whereby the state attempted to conduct the conduct of the medical profession not by regulating the services provided, but by ensuring self-regulation by the profession of entry to its ranks based on an assurance of scientific training. In this way it created a civil space for the self-government of the profession by the profession, minimising the force and ongoing involvement of the state apparatus itself: 'what we have here is, again, a mechanism for a certain "economy" of government; the ideal of the profession as a self-licensing body discloses less the cynical and self-interested project of restricting others from their rights to practise than an attempt to make the act of governing medicine as exact and minimal as possible' (Osborne 1993, p. 348).

The main alternative interpretation is that the profession-controlled regime of medical licensing is a triumph for the upper-class medical profession over other health workers such as nurses, midwives and chiropractors, effected through the class links of the medical profession to governments. Evan Willis (1983) has elaborated this line of analysis in the Australian context in his classic book *Medical Dominance*. Both of these interpretations are useful for understanding the peculiar regulation of the medical profession, and I return to discuss this subject in more detail in Chapter 4 when considering the labour market for medical services.

Setting aside the question of the motivation for the regulation of medical practice, there is another question concerning the effectiveness of such regulation in producing its desired effect, and compliance with such regulation. Braithwaite (Braithwaite, Makkai and Braithwaite 2007) has developed a mid-range theory of regulation in his depiction of a pyramid of regulatory activity. The peak of the pyramid, rarely in action, consists of the statutory power to ruin—professionally or financially—the person or company subject to regulation if they do not comply with the statutory requirements. The middle tier of the pyramid consists of structured inter-actions between the regulators and the regulated that are initiated when there are breaches of regulations, and in which directions are given by the regulator and complied with by the person or company being regulated, with minimal adverse consequences. The base of the pyramid, integral to the daily operation of the regulated field, consists of structured directions and surveillance by the regulator and compliance with directions and co-operation with surveillance by those regulated. In many industries—health included—there is also an even broader base of self-regulation by the industry, without any statutory requirements, but including codes of conduct, standards and accreditation systems and peer review of compliance. Braithwaite and colleagues have found through empirical review that in industries solely regulated by self-regulation or statutes without an apex of tough sanctions for non-compliance, bad behaviour is more common and industry pressures result in frequent breaches and common escalation of regulators' responses to the toughest (but still weak) action available. In contrast, industries where there is a ruinously punitive apex in the system of regulation are characterised by fewer breaches, better co-operation between regulators and those regulated, and industry pressures resulting in more compliance and less need for punitive action, despite there being more and tougher punishments available (Braithwaite, Makkai and Braithwaite 2007). Chapter 7, on quality and safety, shows in more detail how this works in the health field.

Regulation is a way that health considerations can be pursued in sectors outside health care. Much public health policy operates in this way, with statutes regulating the preparation and sale of commercial food (food standards), the water supply, environmental health, chemical use, and so on. This type of regulation may be administered by public health officials in Commonwealth (e.g. quarantine), state (e.g. water) or local government (e.g. restaurants), or by officials in other portfolios (e.g. veterinary chemicals, vehicle safety).

This wider range of regulation to protect public health is a central part of the administration of populations that has developed in the last two centuries. The regulators specified by the health statutes work with the police and the courts to enforce the statutes. Because this enforcement infrastructure is already in place, the marginal cost of regulation is often less to government than the amount of expenditure as incentives that would be required to produce the same effect. However, this comes at the cost of the curtailment of liberty and the risk of producing civil disobedience, and the related dilemmas for the state of how to respond. Civil disobedience by health professionals can often generate extensive public sympathy, making it hard for the government of the day to stick to their policy guns if their democratic majority is under fire.

Where policy about structure is usually thought of as fitting the times and issues to which it responds, policy about regulation is usually thought of in terms of the policy-makers as the universal watchmakers; the regulatory framework is seen as something that will allow the system to run itself, like good clockwork allows the measured unfolding of time to be made manifest without continual tinkering by the watchmaker. Changes to the regulatory scheme are usually thought of as adjustments to the mechanism that will allow it to function without further adjustment.

While such an analysis can be criticised for limiting the policy imagination, it is also a pragmatic approach by a policy community that knows there is limited capacity to sustain an analysis over more than a year or two, so that if a regulatory mechanism is expected to become counterproductive in a few years' time, the chances are that no one then will notice, or if they do will not be placed to reregulate effectively. Regulatory policy feels its historical importance differently than structural policy: regulatory policy-makers feel that they are making history, whereas structural policy-makers feel they are responding to it.

PUBLIC FINANCE FOR HEALTH

Health care is an expensive business, driven by hope and fear, deep science and personal care. Like education, it seems obvious that the government should play a larger role in paying for it. However, a good understanding of the policy arguments about this is important for a very wide range of health policy debates.

This section begins with a brief discussion of how the state raises funds for expenditure on health care, then considers in some detail the arguments about whether the state should intervene in society to raise and allocate funds for health. It concludes with a discussion about the intersection of health financing and fiscal policy. This discussion brings into focus how a lack of recognition of human capital in the accounting rules of fiscal policy creates difficulties for arguments about health financing.

Public financing requires acquisition of funds and the allocation of funds. Usually these transactions are not specifically linked, with money raised being contributed to consolidated revenue and funds for expenditure being allocated from consolidated revenue. For example, the increase in Commonwealth government health expenditure at the introduction of Medicare in 1983–84 was funded by the Medicare levy, introduced as a 1 per cent tax on personal taxable income above the Medicare levy threshold. The revenue generated by the levy goes into consolidated revenue, and is not hypothecated for health spending. It is regarded by the government as the responsibility of the minister for taxation matters (the Treasurer), not the health minister. The levy was increased to 1.25 per cent in the 1987 budget, 1.4 per cent in the 1993 budget and 1.5 per cent in the 1995 budget, but there was no direct link to increases in health outlays. With the increases, the government traded on the goodwill of the public towards the health system and the good name of Medicare to increase personal income tax to meet its fiscal policy objectives.

Occasionally, funds are raised and linked ('hypothecated') to a specific purpose—for example, state governments often charge compulsory service fees for inspection services, and these dollars are used to fund the service itself. Government regulation of health financing—such as the US government's compulsion for employers to buy health insurance for their employees—is similar to hypothecated taxation for health purposes, except that the funds do not pass through government accounts.

A further method of financing health is via tax rebates and tax penalties to encourage purchase of health-related products—for example, health insurance. Interestingly, these rebates and penalties are considered in fiscal policy as income transfers rather than end consumption, and as such are considered to have quite a different effect on national economic performance than government expenditure on health services from consolidated revenue (see below).

In the 1980s, the dominant liberal account of the policy issue of public versus private provision of services relied on the argument that private, market-based provision of services promotes freedom of choice, and that the normal (unfettered) operation of the market ensures the maximisation of public utility (Hayek 1944). In other words, freedom generates value through the market. Within this logic, a theoretical case for public sector provision of services is mounted on the grounds of market failure: that the particular service market in question was not conducive to service providers and consumers freely choosing to contract with each other and therefore the market did not operate to maximise public utility.

The possibility of making a market failure case for public sector expansion rests on a rejection of the assertion that there can be no halfway house between freedom and planning, that the very project of state control over any area of economic activity leads inexorably in the direction of a totally planned society. Following Hayek's Keynesian contemporaries, the Australian National University social theorist Barry Hindess rejects the sleight of hand in Hayek's equation of planning and coercion, along with his rejection of any essentialist account of markets that imbues them with properties (good or bad) not arising from their historical development and the institutional referents that constitute the market and the possibility of exchanges within it:

> there is no necessary opposition between market allocation and public control, and there are numerous ways in which they may combine. What their consequences will be, cannot be determined simply by reference to general concepts of 'the market' or 'plan', but only by reference to the institutional conditions within which they operate (Hindess 1987, p. 146).

It is precisely the historical and structural analysis of the institutional conditions in health system markets that provides the evidence for the market failure argument in favour of the public funding of health care against the fiscal policy orthodoxy. To get into the detail of this, let's now briefly set out the relations between the health service market and the health labour market.

Because the health service market is a service market, its relations to the health provider labour market are particularly important. Three things about the medical workforce are especially determining. First, commencing in the nineteenth century in Australia, state governments put in place medical profession-controlled licensing boards to recognise medical practitioners trained in physical, biological and clinical sciences by universities. Second, the medical profession has undergone a proliferation of specialisations, with the creation of many specialist colleges, faculties and associations, with membership based on postgraduate specialty training programs run by the college, faculty or association. By the 1980s in Australia, the majority of medical practice was carried out as specialist practice; by the 1990s, the bulk of specialist practice in surgery, internal medicine and pathology was carried out as subspecialist practice; by 1995, the Commonwealth government recognised sixteen specialties and 44 subspecialties (termed 'sectional specialties'—NSQAC 1995, p. 8) and only 20 per cent of the medical workforce were vocationally registered as general practitioners. Third, the various specialty bodies control entry to their ranks by operating training schemes to which they control entry as well as by controlling final qualification. Together, these credentialist measures have ensured a medical labour oligopoly to underpin a very strong market position. (For a history of these developments in Australia, see Lloyd (1994) on New South Wales; Willis (1983) and Pensabene (1980) on Victoria; White (1999) on South Australia; and Doherty (1989) and Baume (1994) for later developments.)

Turning to the market for health services proper, the usual economic analysis commences with an enumeration of the features of the so-called ideal competitive market, followed by a list of failures of the empirical health market to achieve this ideal (see, for example, Cooper and Culyer 1973; Mooney 1986; McGuire, Henderson and Mooney 1988; and Arrow 1963 for the seminal review). The ideal is that competitive market pricing integrates the activities of providers and consumers to achieve an equilibrium that is optimally efficient in distributing scarce resources. The features of such an ideal market that are most problematic in the health service market are: the consumer is the best judge of their own desires and understands fully the utility of the service for themselves; there is perfect competition between providers; and externalities (effects on external parties of the exchange between the provider and the consumer) are not significant.

On this account, a free private market for health services is expected to fail to optimise the distribution of scarce resources for several reasons:

- Health care is an unusual commodity in that demand for it is largely derived from the value the consumer places on health, not on health care for its own sake.
- The effect of the health care on the consumer's health is often difficult to predict, requiring both the scientific knowledge and professional judgment of the medical service provider to assess it.
- The medical profession controls admission to its ranks, attempts to control prices (e.g. by the old AMA schedule of fees) and does not allow advertising.

In addition, two externalities are important. First, it is in the community's best interest for people with contagious diseases to be treated to stop the spread of infection, whether the infected person wants treatment or not (the public health externality). Second, many community members wish to see others receive the health care they need, irrespective of the capacity to pay (the caring externality).

In summary, on the one hand in the health sector there is a labour market where, with the support of government (Commonwealth and state), existing providers control entry to new providers through licensing and elaborate training procedures based on the accumulation of scientific knowledge. On the other hand, there is a service market where the major reason for market failure is the information asymmetry between the highly trained providers and the sick members of the public. The anxiety of the public resulting from this asymmetry has been translated into public policy where the government has become a monopsonist purchaser of health services on behalf of the public (a market with only one supplier is a monopoly; a market with only one purchaser is a monopsony).

Another way of summarising the argument is to point out that, without heavy state intervention, the hidden hand of simple markets for health services cannot provide the stewardship necessary to achieve value in the health field. In a sense, this argument demonstrates the need for government stewardship of the health sector in order to assure value from transactions in the provision and financing of health care.

Fiscal policy itself is largely concerned with the overall level of government spending within the total money economy, together with the raising or paying off of government debt and the exertion of a stabilising, counter-cyclical influence on variations in the rate of growth of the national economy. The first budget statement of the Howard government expressed this succinctly as follows:

The Government's medium term fiscal strategy is to follow, as a guiding principle, the objective of maintaining an underlying balance on average over the course of the economic cycle. This approach will ensure that over time the Commonwealth budget makes no call on private sector saving and therefore does not detract from national saving; it will provide the Government with the flexibility to allow fiscal settings to change in response to economic conditions over the course of the cycle and to respond to external shocks (Costello and Fahey 1996, p. 9).

Cross-country comparisons show that health expenditure as a percentage of GDP increases in proportion to the level of GDP per head of population (Blomquist and Carter 1995). Put simply, the wealthier a country is, the higher the proportion of its income it spends on health. This suggests that if Australia's GDP rises over the next decade, the proportion of GDP spent on health will continue to rise. The same effect could also be mediated by the passage of time in response to technological innovations which increase the opportunities for the population to create value by spending money on the pursuit of health.

Under this scenario, the percentage of GDP spent on health would be expected to ratchet up over successive GDP growth cycles. If this is correct—as the AIHW official figures seem to suggest—it introduces the questions of what the expected increase in health expenditure will be spent on, what proportion will be in the public sector and what in the private sector, whether it is possible or desirable for public sector agencies to influence how it is spent and, if so, how this influence should be developed.

A key task of health policy formulators in relation to ideas for health financing is to build into their health policy proposals an understanding of the relationship between the health policy discourse and the fiscal policy discourse. Why should the state spend public money on health at all? How does public expenditure on health care generate greater value in the community than if the money had been left for expenditure on health in the private sector?

The likely impact on the economy of not spending public money on health should be considered—for example, expanded private sector expenditure driven by anxieties but without the health gain that would be delivered by public expenditure. Public sector economists make a policy argument along these lines by noting that leaving such health expenditure to the private sector results in the failure of market mechanisms to maximise the utilitarian benefit from the expenditure because of the inability of consumers to know what they want—or indeed what they are getting—and the vicious cycle of increasing expenditure for no benefit if unregulated insurance and markets develop in an effort to smooth expenditure and spread risk across a group of consumers (Arrow 1963; Ham 2004).

This brings us to another point in the discussion about health expenditure: how it is treated in the national accounts and the Commonwealth government balance sheet. Generally, health expenditure is considered within the national accounts as social benefits within the current account. On the expenditure side of the national accounts, public sector health expenditure is treated as final consumption spending, with the implication that it is a pure drain on national resources, making no contribution to the accumulation of national wealth. This is in contrast to social security payments, which are treated as income transfers, having no net drain on the economy. No health expenditure is treated as a capital transfer (IMF 2001, p. 71). The fiscal policy fashion for restraint causes difficulties for the operation of the health system with its inherent tendency to expansion over time. Conversely, health policy imperatives bring into stark relief the difficulties in fiscal policy orthodoxy around the handling of growth in the service sector and investment in human capital formation.

The separation of expenditure for accounting purposes into consumption in the current account and investment in the capital account developed with respect to the production of goods. The transposition of these categories to accounting for expenditure on services has neglected the formation of human capital, raising a number of questions. Expenditure on building a hospital is considered investment, contributing to the formation of the nation's capital stock. However, expenditure on training doctors to work in the same hospital is considered final consumption expenditure rather than a necessary investment in order to provide a health service out of the hospital. The importance of this is magnified by the fact that the health industry is labour intensive and the health workforce relatively highly skilled compared with most other sectors of the economy of comparable importance (measured in terms of share of GDP).

Going a step further in the health system production process, it is clear that, for some people at least, receiving health services—like receiving education—increases their productivity and can be considered an investment. Clearly, some health expenditure results in a return. For example, influenza vaccination for people in a large office environment results in less influenza, fewer sick days taken and more productivity. Acute care of workplace injuries returns workers to productivity faster and more completely than the natural healing process. Some health measures reduce true health end expenditure in the future (of course, a similar point can be made about food consumption: without it, people's productivity falls dramatically, at least after a certain point). A healthy old age can enable many people to preserve and pass on their capital and reduce the need to liquidate it to pay for their own care and support.

It could be argued that a proportion of national expenditure on the education of the health workforce and on health services should be counted as investment rather than final consumption. If this were done, the national savings ratio would be higher than using current accounting arrangements. Although such an accounting change would not affect the assessment of whether the ratio is adequate to meet national economic policy objectives, the argument could at least be made that these objectives would need to be modified to include targets for future investment in health.

The health sector has a high multiplier due to it being labour intensive, and because it has good linkages to other sectors including education, construction (especially in the current phase of rebuilding the capital stock of Australia's hospital system), manufacturing and high technology. My point here is that the increase in the proportion of GDP spent on health seen with increasing GDP per head of population is in fact contributing to the higher GDP. The logic of this becomes obvious once a proportion of expenditure on health is considered to be investment. The contribution that health expenditure makes to growth in GDP is the return on that investment.

In simplified form, this argument merely states that public expenditure on health services can contribute to an increase in a nation's wealth. This argument was made in England in the 1890s in relation to the health of potential recruits for the Boer War (a crucial part of England's imperialist strategy for wealth creation), and in the Beveridge report (1942) concerning the productivity of the workforce for post Second World War reconstruction. It was made in Australia by the National Hygienists in the first decades of the establishment of the Commonwealth Health Department and the development of Queensland's network of free public hospitals in the 1950s (see Chapter 5).

If health expenditure is going to increase over the next couple of decades, and if the public sector share of health expenditure is to be maintained, these arguments need to be reinvented in relation to the contemporary fiscal policy discourse. The benefit of health gain for the expenditure of public monies on health should also be demonstrated. Economists such as Michael Drummond and colleagues at York University (1980) have made various policy arguments in relation to this, such as that the various options to which public expenditure for health could be directed should be ranked according to their cost/utility ratios, or that the marginal utility of a change in program expenditure should be calculated to value the proposed public expenditure. More recently, the Health Metrics Program of the World Health Organization and the philanthropic investment by the billionaire Larry Ellison in the Harvard-based program to develop a health version of *The Economist* magazine should help bridge the systems of thought of health policy thinkers and economists. However, if this is not done successfully, the consequences could be extensive: a reduction in public sector share of health expenditure; a loss of public policy influence over the development of the health sector; a rapid development of the private health sector; and its divergence from the public health sector in terms of population served and services provided, resulting in a two-tier health system (this is referred to by some commentators as the 'American model') (Williams 1992).

POLICY AND RESEARCH

The relations between policy and research are many and varied. Often they go together naturally and without difficulty. At other times, they can be opposed and cause great difficulties for each other. In some circumstances one may lead and the other be subordinate, or it may be the other way around. Many of these relationships between health policy and research have been excellently laid out by Huw Davies and colleagues at the Research Unit for Research Utilisation, St Andrew's University, Scotland. Three of the higher level relations are that: contemporary governments must justify their support for research; publicly supported research is under pressure to contribute to the public good; and health systems strive to provide care supported by research.

Health services and health policy researchers in Australia and New Zealand are optimistic that their fields of investigation and their close relationship to the stewards of our health system make them well placed to plait these three endeavours (*Journal of Health Services Research Supplement* October 2004). Health services research is well placed to assist in policy formation for a number of reasons. It is often directly relevant to policy dilemmas, because there is more policy about health systems and services than there is about molecular biology or about pathophysiology. There is a high degree of shared culture between policy-makers and health services researchers—personnel move between the two fields, we meet at conferences, and our technical languages overlap substantially. From an epistemological perspective, the limits to the generalisability of health services research, often seen as a weakness by our biological science colleagues, are due to the particularities of culture and the history of health system design. These are precisely the context and circumstance within which policy formation occurs.

Conversely, policy-makers have identified health services research as a field to invest in and nurture. This can be seen in the funding of research to support technology assessment in the Medicare Services Advisory Committee processes, by the work commissioned by the NHMRC Health Advisory Committee through the Guidelines Assessment Register, and by the NHMRC funding for health services research programs.

Yet the gulf remains between the world of the researcher and the world of the policy-maker and health service manager. There is no talking in the library and there are no books in the boardroom: research can tend to be an isolating activity whereas policy and management are subject to a myriad of pressures and demands.

Health research and health policy align on some things and are unavoidably at odds on others. Understanding the relations between the two fields in a pragmatic way may help researchers avoid moralistic posturing and increase their contribution to research translation. It may also relieve some of the exasperation of policy-makers and managers in dealing with researchers, and this may even assist in their stewardship of the research effort itself.

Policy and research activities are practical activities, in some ways related to power and knowledge respectively. Attempts to synthesise an abstract theory encompassing power and knowledge are a recognised philosophical pastime. Power and knowledge are different but bound up with one another: knowledge empowers; power deceives. Perhaps a composite concept combining both with an interesting punctuation mark (e.g. Foucault's 'power/knowledge') can highlight the deception. But if I can generalise, these kinds of abstract syntheses about power and knowledge rarely produce satisfying philosophy outside of theology. The best thinking and writing that spans power and knowledge is about particular powers and knowledge of particular things, and produces particular insights into an important but vexing set of circumstances.

If we were to take a particularist approach to the relations of policy and research, we would examine the activities and relations of researchers in the policy field. We would examine the activities and relations of policy practitioners to research. And we would recognise that these two investigations are quite different: they are not two sides of the one coin—they are almost unrelated. The present discussion emphasises the relation of research to policy, rather than policy to research.

Today's neo-liberal era 'fosters the development of *policy* as the most appropriate form of social problem-solving' (Yeatman 1998, p. 6). There is a normative view, held by many researchers, that the proper process of problem-oriented policy formation, like problem-based learning in medical schools, should mirror the scientific method of identifying a puzzle or knowledge gap: making relevant observations; analysing these to formulate hypotheses; and designing experiments that demonstrate the ability of specific actions to cause certain effects.

Translating this quasi-scientific approach into a policy process then unfolds as follows. A health problem for members of the community is identified as a policy concern. The identification of the problem should be based on sound evidence about the world. Existing research pertaining to the problem should be reviewed, and occasionally additional research commissioned. This research is supposed to provide confidence that certain causes will have certain effects. With this knowledge, effective policy can be made. A corollary is that if research has identified a way to address a social problem, policy-makers should consider adopting it.

This view effectively identifies the scientific method as the normatively preferred way of working out what to do, and is perhaps responsible for the tendency of some researchers to pontificate on how the policy process related to their interests should proceed, despite little knowledge of the practice or history of policy process design.

We should not be surprised that the policy process is not the researcher's strong point. Research is driven by a curiosity to know. This is combined with an expectation that if we know, we will be better off. But we will be better off in ways we cannot know at the time we are planning our investigations (the debate on stem cell research shows this clearly). Knowledge moves in mysterious ways.

The researcher values knowledge for its own sake. The long history of the pursuit of knowledge has seen a shift from the medieval scholastic ethos of acquiring knowledge from authorities, through the empirical turn in the sixteenth and seventeenth centuries towards acquiring knowledge through the experience of experiment, to contemporary scientific practice based on the coordinated activities of a global community of inquirers.

For contemporary scientific practice, with its enlightenment ethos of progress through science, knowledge is king. Turning to the view from the world of policy, the king is king, or perhaps it is the prime minister of Her Majesty's loyal government. If researchers feel they have claim to the normative view of the relationship between research and policy, members of the policy fraternity often feel they can claim the high ground on the practical view of that relationship. On this view, the policy process is subordinate to the politics of government. This includes the 'small p' politics of manoeuvring within the bureaucracies and the 'big P' Politics of the electoral process and the parliamentary parties. The art of the possible, timing and control of the policy agenda, the struggle between interest groups, the formation of coalitions and the accountability for power are felt by the participants to be the primary shapers of the policy process.

From this perspective, researchers proposing a modified scientific method for policy formation can be seen as just one interest group, a view reinforced by the fact that such groups usually call for a policy to be based on their own research, or for more research, or both. In the policy arena, those who claim the truth are regarded as the most dangerous. Further, the policies and policy processes proposed by researchers rarely take sufficient account of the timing, electoral implications or balancing of interests required for getting any sort of satisfactory outcome from a policy process.

Policy in contemporary democratic society reflects our history of power-sharing from the time of the Magna Carta and the development by medieval city-states of a concern with the social security and good order of their citizenry in a way that complemented the aristocracy's feudal concerns with external security. The words 'policy' and 'police' share a common root, from the Ancient Greek word 'polis', now usually translated as city-state. Since the democratic revolutions of Europe and America cut off the king's head, policy has become one of society's principal means for the development of a consensus on what to do together. Democracy operates to create aggregated authority, and this authority underpins the capacity of policy to coordinate action between often very large numbers of people.

Having an appreciation of the different histories of the worlds of research and policy helps us understand the ancient's confabulation of all-knowing, all-powerful god-kings, without whom the gulf between knowledge and power could lead to calamity and despair. How are we secular moderns to bridge this gulf?

We must recognise that policy-making is not a science. Policy often requires the making of decisions in unique circumstances involving large numbers of people. The outcome will not be the long-run average occurrence: it will be a one-off, its outcome knowable only in retrospect. Deciding what to do requires judgment. As John Keane (2004, p. 162) has summarised, 'Judgement, the learned capacity to choose courses of action in contexts riddled with complexity, is among the chief democratic arts.'

The field within which policy operates is communities. These are rapidly changing. Acceptance in the community of the authority of the policy is crucial, and often must be built in quirky, non-repeatable ways. Knowledge can often assist in building such a consensus, and synthesis of research relevant to the policy under consideration can be very helpful. While I do not propose to review how this is best done, I make the observation that the identification by respected researchers of the one or two authoritative scientific articles may have more impact in a policy debate than a comprehensive literature review, because policy debate is about authority.

At a National Health and Medical Research Council (NHMRC) meeting discussing research strategy for the coming three years, a council member with an administration background noted that governments expected council to fund policy-driven research. This came after much discussion about how the council could encourage research-driven policy. A little later, another member, with a research background, remembered the comment in an aside about how cynical governments can be, expecting researchers to find evidence to support policies that have already been made. Of course he missed the point, which was that when governments have made a policy, such as to slow the obesity epidemic or improve co-ordination of care for chronic illness, they should be able to expect, with public funding, that the research community will take up the policy as a challenge and look for the evidence needed to support implementation of the policy. Such policy-driven research questions should be as fruitful in basic science and clinical research as in epidemiology and health services research.

THE ASSEMBLAGE OF THE HEALTH SYSTEM

The health sector comprises around 10 per cent of total domestic economic activity in Australia. It encompasses many activities, institutions, agencies and companies. To make sense of this, it is useful to consider health systems as an assemblage of three main things: management, financing and expertise. These three things are knitted together at all levels of the health system and throughout our health services. Successful health care reform is always about creating new conjunctions of these three things, whether it be the revitalisation of a meandering community health service or the wholesale restructure of a state's regional health services.

At the root of both the information asymmetry in the health service market and the strategy of occupational closure in the health labour market is the constitutive relationship of the health system to scientific medical knowledge. Like all discursive relationships, this relationship is dynamic. Its transformations are intimately related to the transformations of the health system in modern times.

In this section, I outline two historical assemblages of the management, financing and expertise that have shaped the governmentality of health in Australia. The first, the health insurance/clinical services assemblage, emerged in the nineteenth century and has persisted in a relatively stable form to the present day. The second, the funding formula/population health assemblage, emerged in the post Second World War period as a result of a series of major reorientations in the earlier nineteenth century public health assemblage.

In his analysis of the beginnings of modernity, Foucault (1980) has outlined the development of the link between health care and scientific discourse during the eighteenth century, and the implications this had for the institutional structure of the health system at that time—especially the emergence of hospitals devoted to single organs towards the end of the century related to the ascendancy of pathophysiology. This set the scene for the development of the clinical sciences around the pathophysiology of the various discrete organ systems.

Both the discourse of clinical medicine and the discourse of population health have been built into a governmental assemblage within the modern health system. Foucault points in the eighteenth century to:

> the development of a medical market in the form of private clienteles, the extension of a network of personnel offering qualified medical attention, the growth of individual and family demand for health care, the emergence of a clinical medicine strongly centred on individual examination, diagnosis and therapy, the explicitly moral and scientific—and secretly economic— exhalation of the private consultation, in short the progressive replacement (sic) of what was to become the great medical edifice of the nineteenth century (1980, p. 166).

At the beginning of the nineteenth century in France, medical practitioners were licensed by the state to entrench the scientificity of the practice of medicine (Osborne 1993). Similar developments occurred in England and Australia from the middle of the nineteenth century (Willis 1983; Lloyd 1994). This self-licensing regime of medical practitioners led to the expansion of medical practice, mostly organised commercially as individual doctors. It also provided a professional basis for the advancement of medical science as a field of practice. This occurred particularly in the medical schools through which aspiring medical practitioners had to pass to gain a licence. As the profession expanded, its market expanded by the development of insurance arrangements by the bourgeoisie and the petit bourgeoisie. In the nineteenth century, an assemblage of the health system emerged which combined insurance-based funding technology with the clinical sciences to give the distinctive features of the health services systems which have developed in many countries over the last two centuries.

By the end of the nineteenth century, a stable three-part assemblage of the health system had emerged in many western countries, consisting of clinical science, private practitioners and insurance financing. The possibility for the emergence of this assemblage depended on state regulation of both medical practice and private insurance, and the legitimacy for state regulation of these fields derived from their relation to clinical science. This assembly remains in place in Australia today, although its importance within the overall Australian health system has declined since the 1960s.

Technologies of life insurance, workers' compensation insurance and social insurance developed to include payment for doctors' fees (Ewald 1991). Accident insurance, workers' compensation insurance and social insurance covering health costs all reached a state of sophisticated functioning during the nineteenth century in France, Britain and Germany. State intervention in this system began almost as soon as it emerged. This included regulations constraining insurers and reinsurance arrangements, laws obliging insurance to be taken out, and the establishment of authorities to actually run insurance schemes (on the development of insurance technology in the nineteenth century, see Ewald 1991; Defert 1991; for a history of the friendly societies and the development of health insurance in Australia, see Gillespie 1991).

Insurance is a population-based technology in that risk can only be calculated with respect to a population, otherwise insurance would be no more than a wager. Risk only becomes something calculable when it is spread over a population. The work of the insurer is to constitute that population by selecting and dividing risks. As Ewald (1991) has pointed out: 'Strictly speaking there is no such thing as an individual risk; insurance can only cover groups; it works by socializing risks. It makes each person a part of the whole' (1991, p. 203).

The development of insurance was part of the evolution of the bourgeois ethical discourse of the nineteenth century. The initial attraction of insurance as a bulwark against financial catastrophe was linked to a particular moral construction of chance, which was linked to a moral imperative directing the individual to provide against its contingencies. Liberal thought held that whatever nature dealt out was, in itself, just. Chance had to be allowed for, and it was up to each individual to provide against whatever chance might deal out.

The widespread practice of insurance, however, was associated with the emergence of a new conception of justice not attached to chance itself, but to how a group dealt with chance. This concept of justice legitimated the state requiring social insurance arrangements to be made by various groups (guilds, industries) covering welfare and health. Nevertheless, the ethic of insurance retains an imperative oriented towards the individual, at least as the actuarial basis for calculations. The archetype of this was the development of compulsory German social insurance, introduced by Bismark in the 1880s (for a brief account of this, see Appleby 1992, pp. 117–19).

This financing technology was linked to fee-for-service practice by medical practitioners licensed by the state on the basis that their services were carried out broadly within the legitimating framework of the clinical sciences. The state conferred legitimacy on the clinical sciences by procedures for recognising qualified medical practitioners trained in the sciences, and by excluding other health practitioners from access to health care institutions and cover by health insurance (for an Australian history, see Willis 1983). Arrangements within both the financing system and the clinical system had a strong influence over the institutional design of the health system, from the hospitals to the medical societies to the doctors' rooms.

The principal form of aggregation of medical practitioners in the health insurance/clinical sciences assemblage is as a profession, and there are numerous historical accounts of the development and strengthening of the medical profession during the nineteenth and early twentieth centuries (Pensabene 1980). The principal form of aggregation of health care recipients in this assemblage is as a market for health insurance products, including as contributors of data for actuarial calculations.

The institutional structures and traditions of practice that developed around this health insurance/clinical sciences assemblage account for many aspects of our current health system, and it continues to operate actively in the ongoing development of the system. The actual provision of services in this assemblage is essentially a private matter between medical practitioners and patients on a one-to-one basis in a relationship with a style established in ancient times.

In the last few decades in Australia, a new assemblage has emerged in the governmentality of health, combining formula-based funding technology with the population sciences. Following the Second World War, pressure emerged from the public for the government provision of health services—not just their regulation. Public funding for health increased throughout the 1960s, and by the 1970s, with the introduction of Medibank, it was distributed largely to public health institutions or the doctors who worked in them (hospitals, community health centres and the like). During the 1980s, public sector health services had become largely organised into area-based corporate entities. By the early 1990s, the new assemblage could be specified as follows: population science/public health; area-based health services as large public organisations; and public financing by funding formulas.

This new assemblage is on the ascendant as the relationships between the three parts becomes tighter and more complex. The shift towards collective taxation-based financing and population-based service funding has privileged population-based sciences such as demography and epidemiology over organism-based sciences such as pathology and biochemistry. The statistical methods used to calculate funding for populations have become increasingly responsive to medically oriented enumerations of the population, including its mortality, fertility, age and gender structure, and its health service use profile—a useful and direct proxy for morbidity. The importance of public sector health financing has increased in the fiscal policy arena in terms of its increased share of public sector resources. The use of arguments based on population health and health service usage patterns has increased the clarity of arguments for a positive governmental role in financing for the health sector as a crucial, productive part of the national economy.

To summarise, by a decade after the introduction of Medicare, the transformed association of the health system with health science— including the shift to population-based approaches—had reasserted itself as a stabilising influence on the health system in its dynamic development. On the one hand, this relationship facilitates the integration of resource allocation within the health system with knowledgeably defined health need, to bring the morbid anxieties of the public into some kind of balanced contact with the expert practices of health service providers. On the other hand, it secures the flow of resources to the health system by bridging the difference between the discourse on health financing with the discourse on fiscal policy.

This is the latest assemblage of the population health discourse into a health system, the latest particular elaboration of a power politics of health. The insurance/clinical medicine assemblage persists, of course, and has a continuity independent from the formula/population health assemblage. Nevertheless, I would suggest that the new assemblage of public health has not only taken over some of the territory of the old clinical medicine assemblage, but is also ringing in the current changes in the health system. In particular, the contemporary population health discourse has found a new and enthusiastic interest in the financing and operation of public hospitals. On this terrain, it has met up with the clinical discourse in an historically new articulation.

The assumption by the state of the major responsibility for funding health services brought with it two particular pressures. First, it has necessitated the development of central government mechanisms for distributing funds to health service providers. Second, because the funds are collected through taxation imposed by a popularly elected government, the distribution is sensitive to the equity of resource allocations across electorates. These two pressures on the distribution function, combined with a growing concern for allocative efficiency in central government agencies (see Pusey 1991), have resulted in the development of formula-based resource allocation at a number of levels in the health system. Population health sciences inform these formulas, which typically provide funds for region-based health service management. This assemblage is one of the most important arenas for health policy-making in the contemporary politics of health.

4.

GOVERNING DOCTORS

There are probably more laws and statutes governing doctors than for other groups of people in the world. And yet the perception remains that doctors, as a profession, almost always get their way in public policy and, as individuals, can get away with murder. The government of doctors is marked by an enormous number of constraints and breathtaking freedoms. How are we to understand this apparent contradiction?

Taking government to mean the conduct of conduct (Gordon 1991, p. 48) we can consider medical practice to be itself a form of government whereby doctors conduct the conduct of their patients in a pastoral care tradition. At a different level, from the eighteenth century onwards, governments in western liberal democracies have conducted the conduct of doctors through licensing, recognising the autonomy of medical practice as part of civil society, not as part of the state. Since the Second World War efforts to govern medical practice have intensified, with marked shifts in health financing into the public sector.

Contemporary public policy necessarily straddles the government of citizens by the state and the government of patients by doctors. The first part of this chapter outlines the liberal and neo-liberal approaches to coupling the state–citizen style of governing, based on consent, with the shepherd–flock style of governing underpinning medical practice, based on a tradition of pastoral care.

Almost all aspects of health stewardship require a dynamic understanding of the medical labour market. The second part of this chapter provides a brief history of the development of licensing medical practitioners and other health professionals, and a discussion of how this licensing is controlled.

The final part of the chapter goes on to discuss some of the major dynamics at play within the market for professional medical services by considering some of the incentives that influence doctors, particularly a suite of incentives introduced for general practitioners around the turn of the millennium. Of particular interest throughout the chapter (and indeed the book) is the construction of freedom within this field of government. For example, a high value has been placed in Australia on preserving patients' freedom to choose their doctor and doctors' freedom to choose their practice location. The final part of the chapter shows how this value has been mobilised in relation to Australian general practice incentives, in contrast with the more constrained British system.

PASTORAL CARE IN A LIBERAL STATE

Since the late eighteenth century, western governments have attempted to conduct the conduct of the medical profession in a characteristically liberal way. States have sought not to regulate the services provided by the medical profession, but to ensure self-regulation by the profession of entry to its ranks based on an assurance of scientific training. This approach underpinned public confidence in medical services, and provided the basis for an expansion of the market for medical services as a means of improving the public's health. The Australian history of medical licensing is discussed in the next major section. The important feature to note at this point is not the triumph of medical interests, but the specifically liberal character of the licensing approach: what we have here is, again, a mechanism for a certain 'economy of government; the ideal of the profession as a self-licensing body discloses less the cynical and self-interested project of restricting others from their rights to practice than an attempt to make the act of governing medicine both as exact and as minimal as possible' (Osborne 1993, p. 348).

The above description of liberal governance in the health care arena does not sit easily with traditional accounts of government that contrast the ideology of liberalism—including the high value it places on individual freedom—with the practical operation of governments to limit this freedom. Less orthodox, but more useful, is the proposition that the principle of maximum freedom is not the central plank of a liberal ideology, but rather an objective in the administrative technologies of government. In other words, freedom is an idea that, in a very practical way, guides a particular mode of governing. Barry Hindess (1996) describes this analytical shift as follows:

> Liberalism is commonly understood as a political doctrine or ideology concerned with the maximization of individual liberty and, in particular, with the defence of that liberty against the state. However, following Foucault's work on governmentality, a different usage has been suggested, based on the idea of a liberal mode of government. This usage suggests that the sphere of individual liberty should be seen, not so much as reflecting the natural liberty of the individual, but rather as a governmental product (1996, pp. 300–1).

This shift in thinking about liberalism is important. What we now have is not a government which necessarily believes in or respects individual liberty, but rather one which offers it as a product of its administration. This is particularly the case for those areas outside politics, where liberal governments seek to manage without destroying autonomy. Health care is one of those areas outside politics whose existence and autonomy is maintained through the activities and calculations of a proliferation of independent agents, including philanthropists, doctors, hygienists, managers, planners, parents and social workers (Rose and Miller 1992).

A number of writers (e.g. Burchell 1993; Rose 1989; Dean 1991) on the liberal mode of government have argued that this change in liberalism, from an ideology to a 'product', arose with a distinct transformation in the conception of society with which liberal techniques of governing are designed to operate. This transformation is associated with the work of the Chicago School of Economics, Margaret Thatcher's government in Britain, and the Hawke and Keating Labor governments in Australia. The central feature of this transformation, these writers argue, is a changed understanding of the relationship of government to society, and particularly of the relationship between government and market. Burchell (1993) comments that these new liberals differ from earlier forms of liberalism in that they do not regard the market as an already existing quasi-natural reality. Rather, the market exists—and can only exist—under certain political, legal and institutional conditions that must actively be constructed by governments.

From Burchell's point of view, markets are as much a product of government administration as freedom is. Moreover, the work of creating optimum market conditions can now be carried out for the private sector or the public sector in a similar manner: there is no longer any need to see the techniques and rationalisations of government involvement in private sector fields as being fundamentally different from the governmental techniques or rationalisations applicable in the public sector. For the Chicago economic liberals, the model of rational-economic conduct needs to be extended beyond the economy itself, generalising it as a principle for both limiting and rationalising government activity (Burchell 1993, p. 274).

The traditional liberal mentality for governing assumed that it was better for the major spheres of social life—including medical practice—to remain as far as possible outside the state, with exchanges financed by private money. For neo-liberalism (e.g. as represented by the Chicago School of Economics), however, this assumption can be questioned, making it important to ask whether a market arrangement for a set of services like general practice will work better in the public or the private sector, in the sense of optimising the production and distribution of services for greatest community welfare. In Australia (and most OECD countries), this question has been decided in favour of majority state financing of the health sector due to the institutional peculiarities of the health field, particularly the importance of expert knowledge in determining the supply of services and the occupational closure of the medical profession. This acceptance of public sector involvement in a field of social activity such as health services is, however, coupled with a continuing wariness of direct state delivery of services according to a central plan, support for professional autonomy and the development of market-style mechanisms to operate within the public sector.

The confidence engendered by this liberal approach enabled medical practice to continue to develop as a semi-autonomous sphere of government concerned with techniques for governing the health of the public as patients. However, we can contrast the state–citizen model of governmentality, based on consent, with the shepherd–flock model of pastoral power, based on a concern for the welfare of those governed, as defined by those doing the governing. The shepherd provides pastoral oversight of the flock, with a relationship between ruler and ruled that is on the one hand quite intimate and continuous and on the other quite authoritarian. This is different from the relationship between citizen and the agents of a democratic state, based on an idea of a consent-based social contract.

What are the implications of the tradition of pastoral power for the governmentality operating within general practice? The pastoral care model developed in non-state institutions—the church, the boarding school, the medical profession—and much of its ethos was in place before the development of liberalism as an ethos for the governmentality of state institutions from the eighteenth century. Consequently, although the modern form of medical practice has been constituted by liberal mechanisms put in place by governments of state, there is much about it that jars with the liberal tradition of government based on consent in the state–citizen model. The implications of this difference in mentality of government depend on the structure and extent of interaction between state and society. For example, if state and society are considered to delineate quite separate spheres of social activity, the style of governing in each will not be considered a problem from the point of view of the other—at least not a problem to which the governmental techniques of the state should be applied.

In general, government programs directed towards medical care operate as mechanisms of government in a state–citizen field, but have as their objective effects within a shepherd–flock field. On this view, a key thing to understand in policy analysis is how the state–citizen game and the shepherd–flock game are coupled, strange bedfellows that they are. This coupling creates the principal axis of political tension in the design and administrative implementation of governmental programs. In such an analysis, the objective of freedom through policy operation becomes problematised: increasing freedom in one field may constrict it in another. For example, state government aspirations to improve the health of citizens, and the quality of the health care they receive, may interfere with the autonomy of medical practice and produce a dilemma concerning respect for the implementation of liberal principles such as patients' freedom of choice of doctor, and doctors' freedom of choice of practice location, type of practice and even their choice of patients.

The liberal mode of government is defined by its primary concern about matters of freedom, not by the extent of freedom achieved: it problematises freedom as a central issue in the operation of the administrative mechanisms of government. Neo-liberalism offers a particular approach to the design of this daemonic coupling of state game and shepherd game, an approach that is illustrated in the design of the funding programs for general practices introduced during the last decade. Before discussing those programs in more detail below, let's consider the traditional liberalist development of medical licensing in Australia as part of the broader development of professionalisation.

PROFESSIONALISATION AND MEDICAL LICENSING

The general process of professionalisation is enacted in three interlocking dimensions. The very idea of a profession and its position in society—and the medical profession is the archetype—relies on special knowledge, an extensive clientele and freedom to practice. We will now consider each of these in turn.

First, a profession must produce and maintain a body of esoteric generalities or knowledges. These knowledges include empirical understanding of the parts of nature with which the profession engages (people and their natural afflictions in the case of medicine), as well as patterns of reasoning and rules or conventions to guide action. Furthermore, this professional knowledge must require considerable interpretation by a member of the profession for its application in specific circumstances.

Medicine has always been, and the other health professions have at least become, apprenticeship-based in the initial education and training of their members. This secrecy-in-training is well illustrated in the arguments of Hippocrates in ancient Greece, and reflected in the Hippocratic Oath. The actions it prescribes in relation to keeping secret any special knowledge transmitted from teacher to apprentice is one of the main reasons the Hippocratic Oath has fallen into disrepute, and is rarely taken in Australia. Even in the United States, where it retains some popularity, it is often taken in modified form, with a more enlightened approach to knowledge as public good replacing the requirement for secrecy (Markel 2004).

The special knowledges of the medical profession, and health professionals more broadly, have developed over many centuries. The writings of Galen, a Roman Empire writer from the fourth century, were foundational texts for the medieval guilds of apothecaries and physicians and, although not scientific in our modern sense, operated as valuable knowledge for formulating actions thought to improve the health of a patient. The embrace from the sixteenth century of the scientific turn by physicians, who were given a royal charter in England in 1518, and apothecaries, who separated from the grocers company there in 1617 (Peterson 1978, quoted in Willis 1983, pp. 37–8), included the detailed observation and empirical recording of the morphology and tissues of the body and the foundation of modern anatomy and pathology, overturning much of the knowledge that had come down from ancient times. The use of the microscope, invented around that time, greatly accelerated this development of knowledge.

The shift in the laying down of knowledge from an ethos of belief in authority to an ethos of curiosity-driven investigation into the nature of things also fuelled the development of experimental investigations in physiology, with great discoveries such as that blood circulates (by William Harvey in 1616), and that vaccination protects from disease (by Edward Jenner in the 1790s). It was also important that methods of controlled observation could demonstrate that some things could decisively be seen to have no effect, as was the result of King Louis XVI's 1784 royal commission into the (non) effect of Mesmer's fluid, chaired by Benjamin Franklin (Wikipedia on the internet is an excellent starting point for readers who wish to investigate these and other history of medicine topics).

Today, the Australian Medical Council accredits Australian university degrees that educate people for medical practice, and the medical boards of the various states require completion of an accredited degree for registration as a medical practitioner. Such registration is in fact required by state law for people to practise in Australia as a medical practitioner. The practices of medical education itself have emerged as objects of research, and there is a rapidly growing literature on this topic.

The second dimension of professionalisation is reflected in an extensive clientele base. The profession builds this base by extending the range of cases for the application of its knowledge and by competing with or excluding other occupations, perhaps by legislative means, from access to the clients for its professional purposes.

The strategies implemented historically for the medical profession to acquire clientele are extensive. Legislation was passed in Britain in 1838 'to define the qualifications of Medical Witnesses at Coroner's Inquests and Inquiries held before Justices of the Peace' (Sax 1984, p. 13). This legislation applied in the colony of Australia, with subsidiary legislation passed in the same year establishing a voluntary medical register in Sydney. A separate Victorian register was established by further legislation in 1844 (Willis 1983, p. 47).

In 1858, the British *Medical Act* (then also applicable in Australia) established a register for all medical practitioners and set out the qualifications required for registration (Daniel 1990, p. 86). Within two years, this had led to bitter struggles in Melbourne at least, with the *Lancet* reporting 'the very disunited state of the profession as evidenced from a mass of papers and reports in the Melbourne press: indeed, Melbourne and its hospitals have certainly become famous in the annals of social-medical warfare' (*Lancet* 1860, quoted in Willis 1983, pp. 42–3). Occasionally things turned physically violent, with numerous cases of physicians horsewhipping unqualified practitioners in the streets (1983, p. 43). The Victorian Medical Board was established by legislation in 1862 in response to lobbying by the Port Phillip Medical Association (1846–1851, whose constitution predated that of the British Medical Association), the Victorian Medical Association (formed in 1852–1856) and its successor the Medical Society of Victoria, which published a draft act in the *Australian Medical Journal* (begun in 1856) proposing a ban on unqualified practice and compulsory registration of all qualified practitioners (Willis 1983, p. 49) (for the history of roughly parallel events in New South Wales and South Australia see Lloyd 1994 and White 1999 respectively).

James Gillespie's excellent history of medical politics in Australia outlines more contemporary history for the first half of the twentieth century. That period was characterised by tensions between the development of medical services in hospital and private practice on the one hand, and the vision of a wider, coordinated health system with a strong emphasis on preventive public health on the other. The medical profession, mainly organised through branches of the British Medical Association, championed private practice, while state governments, employer associations (particularly in mining areas) and friendly societies organised salaried employment of doctors or capitation contracts to provide care to a defined number of people (Gillespie 1991, Part 1). In Gillespie's view, these tensions played themselves out by the 1940s with 'the defeat of this wider vision of public health and its replacement by policies which concentrated on access to the existing pattern of private health services' (1991, p. xi). This can be seen as a triumph of traditional liberalism in a particular phase of history.

In the decade following the end of the Second World War, fee-for-service medicine was cemented into the Australian health system, mainly due to the urging of the organised medical profession. Private health insurance of the type we know today was first offered in Australia in 1947, modelled on the American Blue Cross insurance schemes. One thousand New South Wales members of the British Medical Association

(BMA) contributed 10 pounds each to establish the Medical Benefits Fund (MBF) (Gillespie 1991, p. 244). MBF policies paid reimbursement benefits for fees paid for medical services, and the fund was backed by the BMA in its struggle to expand fee-for-service practice in contrast to the contract practice linked to the friendly societies. MBF targeted middle income-earning members of the public, and expanded into Victoria in 1952 in association with the Hospital Benefits Association (HBA). This complemented the Commonwealth government's Hospital Benefits Scheme introduced in 1945 by the Chifley government (Gillespie 1991, p. 199) and the Medical Benefits Scheme implemented in 1953 by the Menzies government (Gillespie 1991, p. 265).

In the 1960s and 1970s, there were interesting developments in the separation of medical practitioners into specialists and general practitioners. The distinction between physicians, surgeons and apothecaries predated the creation of the modern medical profession in the mid-1800s, with Edinburgh being the first university to offer joint degrees in physic and surgery. Joint qualifications in surgery and apothecary were already common by then and formed the educational basis of the general practitioner (Willis 1983, p. 38). By the early 1960s, specialist qualifications in surgery, internal medicine and obstetrics required the practitioner to do postgraduate work, usually in the United Kingdom. However, unless the practitioners had independent means or significant patronage, upon their return to Australia most worked in general practice as well as in their specialty, at least until they had established a reputation and often until their retirement.

The specialists, however, had control of the Australian Medical Association (AMA), which succeeded the BMA in 1962. Following the Nimmo Report into the Commonwealth's Medical Benefits Scheme, the Commonwealth, with the support of the AMA, revised the schedule of common fees for various medical services applicable to the Medical Benefits Scheme and to regulated private health insurance fund benefits, so that fees for specialist services increased dramatically, becoming much higher than fees for general practitioner services. The new, higher specialist fees were only paid if the patient had been referred to the specialist by a general practitioner. This was complemented by moves from public hospitals to exclude general practitioners from treating inpatients (a trend that continues in the present, but had largely seen the end of general practitioner access to public hospitals in metropolitan public teaching hospitals by 1975). These measures had the effect of making specialist practice considerably more lucrative, and from the late 1960s most specialists were able to give up the general practice aspect of their work as their loyalty to their patients allowed.

The third element of professionalisation is that members of the profession must maintain freedom to practise within their workplace and within society at large, as well as resisting deskilling and routinisation of their practice (Turner 1987, p. 140).

The above description of the development of specialists shows how the medical profession, as a prototype of the health professions (and perhaps many other professions), mobilised state power to improve the profession's own power in the marketplace. Parsons has argued that this professional power is tempered by health professionals' ethical commitment to their patients. This perspective has a strong historical and empirical basis, no matter how unlikely it may have seemed during some of the more avaricious struggles of the medical profession when changes were introduced to various health schemes in Australia (Gillespie 1991; Daniel 1990).

The acquisition of a statutory base by the medical profession has gone hand in hand with the development of the great institutions of health care: the teaching hospitals; the medical schools; the insurance and benefits schemes; public health statutes giving doctors special powers; and other state programs. Within these institutions, and more broadly, doctors have always struggled to retain professional freedom. They have fought for this freedom against the dictates of employers (e.g. the friendly societies, or hospital managers) and the pressures of competition.

From a practical stewardship perspective, legislation towards the end of the twentieth century to facilitate optimum competition in the Australian economy opened up a new series of policy manoeuvres between governments and the learned medical colleges as state governments have sought to increase their influence on access to specialist licensing and the location of specialist training.

Ironically, the technical freedom so ardently struggled for can only be used in a teleological straitjacket. The professional freedom of the medical profession can only legitimately be used in pursuit of the Enlightenment project of humanity overcoming nature. It may be that this counterpoint goes some way towards explaining the paradox frequently observed between the rhetoric of the AMA emphasising freedom and the militant, somewhat authoritarian actions of this 'prince of trade unions' (Gillespie 1991).

Despite their power as a trade union, doctors still operate within a market, with the government as a major player. The market for medical procedures illustrates some of the dynamic interactions between the financing of health care, the development and control of expertise, and the management of service provision. One example occurs in the private sector for medical services financed by Medicare benefits. A high fee for a particular procedure can lead to a sharp increase in numbers of the procedure, and of the number of doctors performing the procedure, without any appreciable benefit to patients. This is illustrated by the rise of gastroscopies in Australia at around the same time as the discovery by Australia's 2005 Nobel Prize winners, Barry Marshall and Robin Warren, that antibiotic treatment cured ulcers of the upper gastrointestinal tract, thus greatly reducing the potential benefit from examining that part of the body through a gastroscopy.

A second example illustrates the same point, but takes the public hospital sector into the analysis. A different fee for the same procedure paid in different parts of the health care system causes a shift of procedures from the low-paying to the high-paying part, causing industrial difficulties for the former and expenditure increases in the latter. This is illustrated by the different fee paid by the Commonwealth and the state governments for the same procedures through the Medicare Benefits Scheme compared with that paid through public hospitals.

FUNDING FORMULAS AND THE GENERAL PRACTICE INCENTIVES PROGRAM

While financial incentives clearly produce an effect on the activities of doctors, this is powerfully modulated by the professional norms and organisational structures within which doctors work. This can clearly be seen in the operation of a suite of incentives for general practitioners introduced around the turn of the millennium through the Memorandum of Understanding struck between the Australian government, the Royal Australian College of General Practitioners, Australian Divisions of General Practice and the Rural Doctors Association of Australia.

In 1984 the Commonwealth government introduced Medicare, a tax-funded universal health insurance scheme that financed general practice exclusively through fees for services. A decade later, while political support for its broad outline was becoming locked in across the political spectrum, there was considerable policy activity seeking to increase the autonomy of the public hospital sector and introduce competitive management behaviour through regionalisation, formula-based funding and case-mix information systems (Braithwaite 1993a). In tandem with these policy moves, the Commonwealth, in partnership with the medical profession, initiated the general practice reform strategy to improve the allocative efficiency of the general practice market through a variety of program initiatives (GPCC 1992; Macklin 1992).

The General Practice Evaluation Program has encouraged academic research into general practice matters. The creation of divisions of general practice has organised GPs on a geographical area basis. This has provided a way of focusing on the GPs' contributions to the health of the population in the division's area and an institutional structure that has facilitated co-operation between GPs and other services in the area. However, the more significant moves were in terms of funding strategies.

In the latter half of the twentieth century, governments of many western states intensified their longstanding interest in health financing from the regulation of health insurance and moved to actually bring health financing cashflows on to books in public sector budgets. This brought democratic themes to the fore in the subsequent evolution of health financing techniques, including a concern for equity of access to health services and a concern with the quality and efficiency of health service provision on behalf of the (voting) population. It is in this context that funding formulas have emerged as a mechanism for distributing recurrent public sector budget allocations, replete with access to huge services, databases and a calculative logic sensitive to the concerns of democratic government.

With health financing moving into the public sector, the new assemblage emerged based on formula funding, population sciences and larger, area-based service providers with responsibility for the health of a more or less clearly defined population. The formula funding of general practice operates as part of this new assemblage. This new assemblage (including its publicly funded fee-for-service component) shows the hallmarks of the neo-liberal mode of government: it transcends the old distinction between state and market, with public financing being distributed to private practitioners through mechanisms that create market-style incentives within the public financial sector.

The use of formula funding for general practice with the Commonwealth's Practice Incentives Program (PIP) in the 1990s was an important event in the development of technologies for governing health in Australia. As a case study, it provides an opportunity to reflect on the intersection of the liberal mode of government and the health system, particularly general practice.

In response to governmental pressures that developed in the wake of the shift of health financing to the public sector, the government identified the desirability of a blend of payment techniques for financing general practice. The Practice Incentives Program, initially called the Better Practice Program, was introduced in 1994 and evolved into the Practice Incentives Program in 1999. In this historical context, the PIP can be seen as part of the recently emerged assemblage in the government of health comprising public sector funding (often involving formulas for its distribution), population science and area-based practice with a population focus. The PIP formula itself includes a patient numbers variable not sensitive to service volume, a patient continuity variable which rewards doctors for their patients' loyalty, and a rural loading. Each of these terms can be understood as mechanisms that provide the benefits of a patient enrolment/capitation payment system (as used in the United Kingdom) without the restrictions on patient and doctor freedom inherent in that system. The PIP also uses eligibility criteria, stating that:

- the practice is a bona fide general practice in good standing (i.e. where the practitioners have not been involved in fraudulent practices or faced disciplinary procedures from a medical registration board);
- 90 per cent of services are provided by recognised GPs (the HIC recognises GPs involved in continuing education on advice from a committee constituted by the Commonwealth Department of Health with representatives from the RACGP and the AMA);
- the practice offers continuity of care between the doctors in the practice, in particular through shared patient records;
- the practice provides a comprehensive range of services, including out-of-surgery visits where necessary and an emergency service 24 hours a day; and
- the practice provides a practice information sheet and undertakes regular patient satisfaction surveys.

In general, the eligibility criteria have been drawn from standards developed by the Royal Australian College of General Practitioners (RACGP) for practice accreditation (RACGP 1993). The criteria are not onerous, and are met by around 95 per cent of the practices that apply. The PIP program also includes incentives for accreditation, computerisation, care planning, health assessments of the elderly, teaching medical students, practising in a rural area and cervical screening. Some of these incentives were associated with rapid increases in the relevant activity (e.g. accreditation of general practices, computerisation of some clinical work and student teaching) and some have had a delayed effect on doctor activity that has been mediated by cultural and organisational change (e.g. care planning).

An important aspect of the PIP program is the administrative mechanisms that are used to affect medical practice in ways that are in accord with the ideas of neo-liberalism. In the first instance, it should be noted that PIP is a publicly funded program that attempts to influence the conduct of general practice by providing financial incentives. As a consequence, the marginal changes that occur as individual practices seek to maximise their share of available PIP funds are expected to contribute to the optimisation of the effectiveness and efficiency of general practice in aggregate. Moreover, in stark contrast with the financing of general practice in the United Kingdom, the PIP eschews command-style administrative mechanisms and adopts a quasi-market approach. As such, the PIP acknowledges and promotes the freedom of choice of doctors and patients in relation to the particular behaviours it is concerned with governing.

In more general terms, the use of a formula to distribute funds with inbuilt incentives for service providers is an innovation in program-based expenditure that links policy objectives to output measures in a highly dynamic way. It has low marginal transaction costs because input data for the formula are already largely available.

The remainder of this section gives a more detailed view of the emergence of the PIP in the blended payment strategy in response to pressures within the prevailing fee-for-service system. It is at this level of analysis that the micro-physics of power can be understood in the neo-liberal mode.

As discussed further in Chapter 8, in 1983–84 the recently elected Commonwealth Labor government nationalised health insurance for medical services, using an approach based on the by then-defunct Medibank scheme introduced in 1975. It made private insurance for medical services illegal, introduced its medical benefits scheme which extended benefits from the pre-existing means-tested scheme to cover all permanent residents, and introduced a new flat tax (the Medicare levy) to cover the increased cost to government of these reforms. Despite the inherently socialist feel of this strategy, the Medicare Benefits financing system for general practice introduced can be interpreted as having a number of neo-liberal features.

On the positive side, in a fee-for-service system all GPs receive from the government (via their patients) the same amount for the same service rendered (notwithstanding that only vocationally registered GPs can access certain items, or arguments about the appropriateness of the fee schedule). This gives the program a perception of fairness in line with the equal pay for equal work principle. This encourages GPs to see all patients who wish to consult them, and has helped to better distribute doctors to practise in poorer communities. Because the time tiering of service items rewards shorter consultations at a higher hourly rate than longer consultations, it also provides an incentive for GPs to deal with patients in a timely fashion, and to recall patients for follow-up consultations. It has also allowed special interests to develop in general practice, such as women's health, men's health, sports medicine, acupuncture and geriatrics, with a certain amount of this practice being on referral from other GPs. The Medicare Benefits program for financing general practice openly embodies the ethos of equality of treatment common to state–citizen administrative arrangements. Concerning the doctor–patient relationship, it aims to remove any financial duress from the part of the patient and thus improve access to general practice services. This has been achieved with considerable success. The schedule of services also affects the style of practice so as to enhance throughput efficiency.

There have also been a number of unintended consequences. While the general design of Medicare has no doubt led to significant efficiencies in the general practice part of the health system, it also provides incentives to save time by outsourcing diagnostic and procedural work through referral to other doctors. As these have become two of the most rapidly developing fields in contemporary medical practice over the last decade, this may have contributed to deskilling in general practice, especially in relation to other fields of medicine. In other words, the Medicare Benefits program may have exacerbated the constriction of general practice within the broader field of medical practice and led to structural inefficiencies in the form of increased number of cross-referrals, consequently increasing costs to the health system as a whole.

All parties represented in the Commonwealth parliament support Medicare and the availability of bulk billing by the doctor for patient Medicare benefits where no patient copayment is charged. The mainstream interpretation of this is that they support a tax-financed, comprehensive health insurance system with free access to public hospitals, and publicly financed, free-at-point-of-service community-based consultations with general practitioners (and specialists on referral) where both the doctor and the patient agree. At the time of writing, around 80 per cent of GP consultations were bulk billed.

The fee-for-service benefit financing system was adopted from the private health insurance system it replaced as part of the minimalist approach to establishing a publicly funded health system. However, the longer the Commonwealth government retains the lion's share of responsibility for financing general practice, the more the imperative asserts itself for the Commonwealth government to develop the range of programs with effects on general practice. All programs are limited in their scope of effect, and have unintended consequences arising from their core elements, which are thus not amenable to alleviation by adjustments to that program. A set of programs utilising a variety of administrative technologies, and concerned with both financing and professional practice issues, has the potential to allow a broader range of government objectives in the field of general practice to be formulated and pursued. This approach also allows the alleviation of unavoidable unintended consequences on one program through the operation of another. This was noted in the National Health Strategy Issues Paper on the future of general practice in its discussion of the proposal to blend fee-for-service with capitation, salary and sessional payment mechanisms: 'The four main payment options all have their strengths and weaknesses, but they can be "blended" to take advantage of the strengths while cancelling out undesirable features' (Macklin 1992, p. 121).

Since the introduction of Medicare, specialist medical practice has been financed through a blended payment system, including Medicare Benefits and state government health system remuneration mechanisms. These include sessional payments, salaries, retainers and honorary (a mixture of barter and altruism) financing approaches, all of which are linked to an active interest in the style of practice in the public hospital system. General practice was unusual in having only one Medicare financing stream, through Medicare Benefits. The development of the Commonwealth government's General Practice Strategy from Brian Howe's period as health minister (1990–93) sought to diversify funding mechanisms into a blended payment system at the same time as increasing the government's interest in other (non-financial) aspects of general practice such as development of the scientific knowledge base, integration with the rest of the health system, improving standards of practice and encouraging a more even distribution of GPs throughout the population.

In the microeconomics of general practice, a distinction can be made between fixed and variable practice costs. Fixed costs include rent of premises, fit-out costs, employee salaries and continuing education. Variable costs include consultation-related consumables and the doctor's time in consultations. Within a blended payment system, Brian Howe put the argument that the government should ideally change its general practice financing mechanism to fund variable practice costs with a fee-for-service system related directly to the throughput of the practice, and fund fixed practice costs on a quarterly payment basis related directly to the total number of patients being cared for by the practice. This would give government a focus on population-based funding of general practice, offer increased leverage over the distribution of practices throughout the population compared to a largely fee-for-service system, and provide a clear basis for the government to take an interest in aspects of general practice other than those relating to patient throughput (such as premises, after-hours availability and equipment levels).

The concerns of government were echoed in consumer consultations held to discuss general practice reform. Broom (1991) found that consumers would support a shift from the fee-for-service system to address quality concerns: 'Consumers identify the fee-for-service method of remuneration as containing incentives that do not encourage quality care. They believe that the options of practice grants, contracts, and salaried arrangements could address some of these concerns' (1991, p. 1). This research showed that consumers would support new financing arrangements that facilitated a health care partnership with their doctor focused on promoting health (e.g. see Cumming et al. 1989) rather than the emphasis on fees for treating occasions of illness (Broom 1991).

The blended payment strategy allows a neo-liberal rationality to be elaborated in relation to general practice. This strategy seeks to draw GPs into the governmentality that arises from the public sector financing of general practice in the Medicare era. The National Health Strategy posed a question concerning 'government as regulator, as payer and planner—what capacity is there for GP input?' (Macklin 1992, p. 32). The answer was essentially that there was very little, but there should be more. As the Commonwealth government, with its increased role in health financing, has increased its interest in goings-on within the shepherd–flock issues of clinical care, so conditions have developed supporting greater involvement of GPs in citizen–state issues of health policy, such as access of patients to general practice and cost control across the health budget. The Commonwealth's general practice strategy promotes an intensified form of government of general practice, whereby 'relations are established between various centres of calculation and diverse projects of rule—more or less "rationalized" as the case may be—such that events within the microspaces of . . . [the] medical consulting room might be aligned with the aims, goals, objectives and principles established in political discourse or political programmes' (Rose 1993, p. 287). This is a process that many GPs are expected to resist, as expected 'professional groups will bargain, bicker and contest on the basis of different claims and objectives instead of meshing smoothly and with complete malleability in the idealised schemes of a programmatic logic' (Rose and Miller 1992, p. 190).

This is the contest of government: debating how to conduct the conduct of GPs. The achievement in reforming the government of general practice is not so much the current suite of programs, but the creation of a centre for the government of general practice in the Commonwealth Health Department in the early 1990s, expanding to a Primary Care Division by 2004, including the extensive consultative structure and the cash flows that have been established.

This Primary Care Division, through its strategic planning, its assessment and funding of clinical divisions of general practice across Australia, and its use of Medicare claims and other systematically collected data to calculate incentive payments to GPs, greatly enhances the capacity for conducting the conduct of general practice. It does this in a decidedly liberal manner which recognises and encourages the autonomy of GPs. It also continues the operation of a market for GP services where providers and consumers can position themselves and freely choose one another (this is discussed in more detail below) and employs the collegial style of organisation preferred by the medical profession. At the same time, it recognises the role in health system steerage accorded to the Commonwealth through its continued control over health financing.

NEO-LIBERALISM IN GENERAL PRACTICE FINANCING

The first payments through the PIP formula were made in early 1995. By January 1996, some 38 per cent of practices were receiving a quarterly PIP payment averaging $11 400 per participating full-time GP, a total of $50 million a year, which was 6–7 per cent of Medicare benefits paid to those practices and probably around 5 per cent of total general practice financing in Australia. Funding formulas for public sector program expenditures have evolved out of recurrent budget processes (for the classic review of this process, see Wildavsky 1979) as a technique for rationally formularising resource allocations to service providers in an attempt to dampen political problems arising from the annual round of competing claims on a limited program budget.

In the evolution of public sector managerial techniques, funding formulas have incorporated performance indicators into their calculations so that the total amount of the payment varies according to how the funded agency performs according to the indicators used in the calculation. This reflexive variability according to specified policy objectives has replaced ad hoc variability according to annual budget round negotiations. Thus formula-based resource distribution mechanisms can provide an impartial basis for resource distribution from a single funder to multiple service providers, and facilitate the development of internal markets in service systems fully funded by the public sector.

In economic terms, a formula for funding general practice, such as the PIP formula, is a public sector, non-price-based resource distribution mechanism linked to consumer choice of GP services. Butler (1994) has rehearsed the argument that the conditions required for an unfettered market price-based rationing system to maximise community welfare are clearly not met in relation to general practice services (1994, p. 20). In particular, supplier-induced demand operates in the exchange of GP services (1994, pp. 26–7) which, given the information asymmetry that characterises these exchanges (Arrow 1963), may not be inappropriate.

In markets like this, a quality-sensitive central distribution mechanism (such as the PIP formula), which provides incentives for supplier-induced demand of particularly valuable services, could improve community welfare where price signals fail to do this. In this scenario, clear policy objectives and formula-based mechanisms to translate them into effective incentives become one of the keys to an efficient (albeit fettered) market system. Against this view, there is evidence that general practitioners do not respond very much to incentives in any form, and the pessimistic possibility that, if they did: 'In the end carrots and sticks may make general practitioners behave more like donkeys than doctors' (Harris 1994, p. 74).

Clearly, how we pay for health does matter. But through the implementation of the general practice strategy since 1991, with its encouragement of a variety of payment systems, the Commonwealth government has articulated a set of financing mechanisms that also address non-financial health policy objectives (Macklin 1992, pp. 121–2). This represents the neo-liberal 'daemonic coupling' of state–citizen and shepherd–flock games discussed above.

Non-formula-based payments to general practices were introduced in 1991, and have included demonstration project grants paid directly to general practices (until 1994), project grants through divisions of general practice and the Rural Incentives Program grants. Formula-based payments were suggested by a joint committee of the Commonwealth Department of Health, the College of General Practitioners and the Australian Medical Association. They were to be linked to an accreditation system so that 'accredited practices be entitled to apply for an annual practice enhancement payment. These grants would be based on a formula, to be developed, but may include factors such as the size and location of the practice and the level of accreditation attained. A weighting for isolated or rural practice might also be added' (GPCC 1992, p. 8).

To summarise the administrative arrangements, the government introduced the PIP as a new general practice financing mechanism in late 1994, with three key features. First, payments are made to general practices (not individual GPs), as an additional source of income to fees for services. Second, practices wishing to receive the PIP payments must satisfy various eligibility criteria concerning the nature of the practice, the information it makes available to the public and the services it provides. Third, payments are calculated according to a formula that takes into account the number of patients seen by the practice, their loyalty to the practice and whether the practice is in a rural location.

Each of these features is intended to have an effect on the governmentality of the field of general practice care. The payments are intended to improve the coordination of services between GPs within a group practice, through such things as common medical records, cooperative after-hours arrangements and patient satisfaction surveys covering the whole practice. This operates through the eligibility criteria but also through the formula itself: where not all doctors in a practice join in the application for a PIP payment, the applying doctors are seriously penalised through the operation of the continuity variable. The payments are intended to provide an incentive for doctors to encourage patient loyalty—more technically, to maximise the proportion of a patient's total GP services that their practice provides. They also provide a separate incentive for GPs to establish practices in rural Australia, where GP-to-population ratios have traditionally been lower than in the cities.

Of course, the factors positively associated with a higher PIP payment are not the only factors which are associated with 'better' practices. In fact, some styles of practice usually considered valuable are actively discouraged by the incentives in the PIP formula, bringing its fairness into question. For example, practices which offer extended hours of opening and see patients from other practices after hours, or which have a well-developed special clinical interest recognised by other practices, may effectively be watering down their continuity index. Although these aspects of better practice are recognised in the entry criteria for the PIP, they could thus be penalised in the operation of the formula. This is an expected situation within the blended payment strategy, and it can be argued that this undesirable feature of the PIP formula is cancelled out by the positive rewards through the fee-for-service revenue generated by these practices.

FREEDOM AND THE DESIGN OF THE PRACTICE INCENTIVES PROGRAM

Finally, let us look in more detail at the objectives of the PIP in comparison to the UK system of patient enrolment/capitation payment. In policy discussion on how to structure a blended payment system, there was considerable interest in a patient enrolment system linked to simple capitation grants (Veale and Douglas 1992, p. 32; Macklin 1992, p. 112). On the face of it, an enrolment/capitation system could have delivered improved patient loyalty, reduced the emphasis on maximising the number of services per patient and been used to achieve better distribution of practices—all central objectives of the PIP—far more effectively than the formula system eventually chosen. My argument here is that the decisive advantage of the formula approach lies in its superior administration of freedom, a feature of great value for the prevailing neo-liberal mode of government.

There is considerable evidence that, other things being equal, greater patient continuity in general practice is related to various indicators of quality of care, including improved management of chronic conditions, less frequent occurrence of harmful incidents, reduced use of resources and improved opportunities for health promotion (Commonwealth DHS&H 1995). Conversely, concern has also been expressed that discontinuity of care leads to higher costs and worse outcomes (Douglas 1991, p. 14; Douglas and Saltman 1991, p. 26), despite the difficulties in actually demonstrating these links (McCallum et al. 1995, p. 2). There are also a number of other important associations with higher continuity, including rural practice location, higher patient socioeconomic status, lower GP service use and lower incidence of bulk billing (McCallum et al. 1995, Table 4; Rosenman and Mackinnon 1992, p. 419). McCallum's analysis is based on data concerning individual GPs, not practices. Nevertheless, it raises the possibility that practices which bulk bill most patients, whose patients are worse off and need more services, get lower PIP payments in association with this.

In the United Kingdom, free choice of doctor was promoted by the government in reaction to the friendly society system in the establishment of the panel system in 1911—a system preserving, for example, the principle of free choice of doctor (Osborne 1993, p. 352). After the Second World War, the United Kingdom introduced the National Health System in which GPs were contracted to provide services within a specific area with payment being made on a capitation basis—a funding formula determined almost solely by how many people were enrolled with that practice. This system provides only very limited choice of GP to patients, and severely restricts the opportunities for GPs to set up practice. It must be recognised that the circumstances of the introduction of this system differed markedly from the circumstances of the introduction of the PIP.

In Australia, the friendly society system gave way to a system of health insurance, introduced by doctors in the successful campaign to stop the establishment of a nationalised health system in the post Second World War period (Gillespie 1991). This health insurance system has never specified that a benefit will only be paid for services from a particular GP. When Medicare was introduced, private health insurance for general practice services was made illegal by the Commonwealth government. Instead, a government benefit was paid to patients, irrespective of their choice of GP.

Freedom of choice of GP was thus built into the government regulation of private health insurance, in the means-tested benefits system prior to Medibank, in Medibank (introduced in 1975, see Scotton and MacDonald 1993), and in Medicare. It has been a cornerstone of the way in which the Commonwealth government has administered the health system in the postwar period, and can be interpreted as realising the government's inclination to interfere as little as possible in the marketplace for medical services, restricting its involvement to financing and not seeking to regulate patient choice of doctor or doctor choice of practice location.

The PIP formula operates to provide the benefits within the shepherd–flock game of general practice that are delivered by the enrolment/capitation system of health financing, at the same time overcoming the limitations to personal freedom inherent in that system. One of the advantages of a patient enrolment/capitation system is that it discourages unnecessary provision of services, as the final payment is not dependent on the volume of services provided but on the number of patients enrolled. Without pursuing the option of patient enrolment, the practice size variable of the PIP formula provides a non-volume-dependent payment function based on patient numbers and share of total care provided: unlike fee for service, the formula payment does not depend on the volume of services provided to each patient. This aspect of the PIP formula accounts for probably the greatest portion of the variance in PIP payments between practices.

The unproven capacity of a system of incentive payments—contributing an average of only around 10 per cent of the public sector income of participating practices—to produce effects on patient loyalty contrasts with the UK system of patient enrolment in a single general practice in that country. Under that system, patient loyalty—or perhaps we should say patient capture—is virtually guaranteed. As mentioned above, this approach was considered for Australia, but this line of thinking was abandoned following the finding that the majority of focus group participants in a well-conducted qualitative study had reservations about being required to enrol with a general practice (AGB Australia 1992a, p. 18), and that in any case 80 per cent of GP users report visiting only a single practice in a given year (AGB Australia 1992c, p. 3). This comparison underscores the Australian government's commitment to maintain the extra degrees of freedom available in the Australian general practice field compared with the United Kingdom.

Another advantage of the enrolment/capitation system is that it can be administered to ensure an even distribution of GP-to-patient ratios across the country. In the Australian context, there is a much lower ratio of GPs to population in rural Australia than in urban areas. In the 1980s, a governmental policy objective was established to encourage redistribution of GPs from urban to rural areas, and this objective underpins the Rural Incentives Program established in 1990. The rural loading in the PIP formula provides a further incentive for rural general practice without resorting to patient enrolment as a tool to control doctor:patient ratios.

With the PIP, the diversification of general practice financing into a blended payment system has been achieved, and it carries the implementation of several of the government's key objectives for the microeconomic reform of general practice. The value of the PIP is not only its capacity to improve patient loyalty by electronic prescribing or encourage doctors to move to rural areas and so on, although these things are valuable achievements. These explicit policy objectives are the acceptable clothing for a muscular additional technology of government. The primary significance of the PIP is that a new set of public sector financial incentives has been instituted for governing general practice.

The formula mechanism of the PIP is a powerful administrative technology that could prove attractive for introducing a range of new policy objectives which could be articulated by the new government. Possibilities include: the creation of a national general practice clinical data exchange with practices which contribute data rewarded by an e-health term; the development of outcome measures for general practice contributions to further national health, with a new health outcomes term based on these measures; and a reduction in general practitioner referrals to specialists, with the money saved redistributed through a self-sufficiency term. All of these possibilities would rely on the PIP formula to provide incentives to GPs to make choices which, in aggregate, would support the policy objectives.

In summary, the PIP is an innovative development in the financing of general practice. The funding formula that is its key mechanism confers on the program a neo-liberal administrative character and has considerable potential to carry further policy objectives. The neo-liberal mode of government is concerned with improving the effectiveness and efficiency of government outlays in meeting defined policy objectives. In this context, Commonwealth policies and programs that conceptualise general practice services as a market can be used to develop powerful leverage over the field because in market terms the Commonwealth is a near-monopsonist purchaser of general practice services. The PIP formula puts a value on GP activities which relates to its policy objectives, legitimated with reference to improving population health, and differentially remunerates GPs accordingly. The general practice profession, as a loose cartel of general practice service providers, predictably resisted this development initially, but embraced it when given the opportunity to participate in detail in the design of the incentives. This neo-liberal administrative play allows the Commonwealth to intensify the government of general practice through a mechanism that is responsive to the traditional liberal value placed on public and professional freedom in the field of general practice.

5.

PUBLIC HOSPITALS AND PUBLIC HEALTH

Hospitals, and more broadly systems of hospitals, are very stable institutions. They change, of course, but they change slowly and the dynamics of that change are carried on long rhythms. This makes a sense of history particularly important for analysing the present states of play in hospital reform. As citadels of the health professions—the medical and nursing professions in particular—the history and dynamics of these professions must also be understood. In addition, the Australian hospital system is very big: it accounts for perhaps 4 per cent of the total domestic economy in its immediate expenditures (AIHW 2006).

In the last 20 years, there has been a profound change in the way Australian hospitals are funded by governments. Most Australian states have organised their hospitals into area-based collections, (area health services in New South Wales, health care networks in Victoria), which also include non-hospital service agencies such as community health centres. These areas are now generally funded according to a formula which divides available monies between the various areas or networks.

The incorporation of acute hospital funding into a formula calculated according to population size invites the elaboration of population health ideas in relation to acute hospital services. Until the middle of this century, despite some shared history, the organ-centred discourse of clinical medicine had few points of articulation with the population-centred discourse on public health. The recent meeting of these two discourses in the hospital, brought about in part by the introduction of population-based funding formulas, is an event of long-term significance for Australia's hospital system. This chapter opens up an analysis of this event.

In order to situate this conjunction of hospitals and public health in its historical context, Foucault serves as an authoritative historian of medicine and health systems, and provides a starting point for analysis. Foucault has produced histories of pathophysiology, of clinical diagnosis (Foucault 1973), of psychiatry and psychiatric hospitals (Foucault 1971) as well as of community hospitals (Foucault 1980) and a naval hospital. His three-volume *History of Sexuality* (Foucault 1976, 1986, 1988) has also been very influential in the development of the theoretical basis for understanding the global HIV/AIDS pandemic. In Volume 1 he coins the term 'biopower'. Broader than the concepts of 'manpower' in the economy or 'firepower' in defence, biopower is perhaps the main field of action for the politics of state. Referring to the individual and population dimensions of biopower, he suggests that the governments of modern society developed between two poles: on the one hand, the anatomo-politics of the body with its accompanying disciplines; and on the other, a biopolitics of the population with its accompanying regulations and enumerations.

This chapter is an analysis of biopower in relation to the hospital. It begins with some history about the study of biology, and shows how this relates to the origins of modern clinical practice. Then, drawing on the work of Ian Hacking and others, the origins of modern population health practice are discussed and some historical points of articulation between these two discourses are noted. The chapter then describes two assemblages in the governmentality of the health system as a structural model for under-standing the contemporary health system. These assemblages consist of scientific knowledge, health service delivery and financing technologies brought into relation with each other. This is followed by a discussion of developments over the last few decades in hospital financing, including moves towards global budgeting and formula funding, using the intro-duction of a Resource Distribution Formula in the New South Wales health system during the 1990s as an example. I argue that the funding formula regime helps forge a therapeutic alliance between the clinical and population health discourses.

THE ORIGINS OF MODERN HOSPITAL MEDICINE

Foucault's histories are concerned with the construction of knowledges and the operationalisation of these knowledges in technologies of power.

In *The Order of Things* (1990a) he describes the transformation in the construction of knowledges about three empirical spheres of society (money, life and language) towards the end of the eighteenth century, in an attempt to lay out the fundamental presuppositions of knowledge in the modern period. Our interest here is in his history of the life sciences.

The Order of Things begins by describing a medieval system of knowledge (what he calls an episteme) based on similitude—on concepts of emulation, analogy and sympathy mobilised in descriptions of 'the prose of the world' (Foucault 1990a, Ch. 2). He gives an example from Crollius (1624) noting 'the affinity of the walnut and the human head: what cures "wounds of the pericranium" is the thick green rind covering the bones—the shell of the fruit; but internal head ailments may be prevented by use of the nut itself "which is exactly like the brain in appearance". The sign of affinity, and what renders it visible, is quite simply analogy' (Foucault 1990a, p. 27).

This gave way in the seventeenth century to an episteme of rationally ordered resemblances, and to knowledges based on representation. The table of knowledge was the archetypal form of this representation; the system of Cartesian coordinates perhaps its most pure expression (Foucault 1990a, Ch. 3). During the eighteenth century, natural history developed as a classificatory—specifically a taxonomical—science that sought to tabulate the forms of nature. Organisms were classified according to morphological characteristics using a method of description, comparison and identification of resemblances. Buffon's system was the best known of these. A more sophisticated taxonomy was developed by Linnaeus which systematically classified life-forms according to some predesignated natural function, such as 'all the different parts related to fructification' (Linnaeus, quoted in Foucault 1990a, p. 140) with the classification then depending on variables of form, number, arrangement and magnitude. Through the episteme of resemblance, nature could be read systematically: the system of signs in the classical age was identical with the order of things. 'The natural order is formulated in a theory that has value as the correct interpretation of the real series or table: moreover, the structure of beings is both the immediate form of the visible and its articulation' (Foucault 1990a, p. 205).

Against the background of this system of representation and the rococo elaborations that it produced within the taxonomia, Foucault sought to 'characterise the mutation that occurred in the entire western *episteme* towards the end of the eighteenth century' (Foucault 1990a, p. 206).

The social construction of the nature of knowledge was transformed by a fundamental reorganisation of the relation between how things were seen and how they were talked about.

Here we have one of Foucault's most interesting historical insights: he traces the folding of knowledge about the table of representation into the empirical ground of the table itself. The description of the system of knowledge that frames the representation of things gives way to a search for the internal principles of the variability of things, resulting in a proliferation of new knowledges: organic functions in the case of biology; capitalist production in the case of political economy; and the principles of the internal generation of phonetic and syntactical regularities in the case of philology. The internal principles of variability are expressed in the *genetic* structure of tables, recasting the relations of knowledge expressed in the tables to their external referents in the world:

> This space [of knowledge] has now been dissociated and as it were opened up in depth. Instead of a unitary field of visibility and order, whose elements have a distinctive value in relation to each other, we have a series of oppositions: they are no longer of the same fabric, they are no longer established in relation to each other on a homogenous surface: the differences proliferate on the surface but deeper down they fade, merge and mingle, as they approach the great, mysterious, invisible focal unity, from which the multiple seemed to derive, as though by ceaseless dispersion (Foucault 1990a, pp. 268–9).

This internalist approach to the production of knowledges marks the close of the classical age and the beginning of modernity in the late eighteenth and early nineteenth centuries. The baton of leading scientific discovery passed from the taxonomists and their elaborate tables to the new biologists and their internal principles, which played a similar role in biology as the laws of the universe did for the physicists from Newton's day.

For the taxonomists, the relative importance of the various organ systems was related to their value for generating taxonomies. The organs could be read as playing a role in life or having a function for the organism. But the taxonomists' reading of function was superficial, and relied on the same mode of decipherment as the description of characteristics concerned with identification and the establishment of a relation to other organisms. By contrast, the new biologists gave central prominence to function. The form of the organ is now read as an expression of biological' function. The interrelatedness of the various functions of the organism lies at the heart of this conception, the actual morphology and its variation being just an expression of this. The discovery and classification of functions and their interrelations becomes the task of modern science. The classification of organisms was to be subordinated to this new principle. Where Linneaus's taxonomy worked particularly well for plants—because their organs are exposed externally; spectacularly in the case of the organs of reproduction, namely flowers—the new biology made speedy progress in relation to the animal kingdom: 'Animal species differ at their peripheries and resemble each other at their centers; they are connected by the inaccessible, and separated by the apparent. Their generality lies in that which is essential to their life; their singularity in that which is most accessory to it' (Foucault 1990a, p. 267).

For the taxonomists, the principles of the construction of knowledge derived from the ideal requirement of the table of living beings that it be read directly from nature. For the new biologists, the principles for the construction of knowledge derived from the invisible functions of the organ and the organism. Classificatory principles expressed in the ordering of things give way to genetic principles expressed in the forms of life themselves. The articulation of these functional principles has been separated from the attribution of form to function, and thus the space of modern biological knowledge has been opened up.

The new biology was profoundly significant for the development of medicine. Indeed, Foucault had earlier addressed the theme of its emergence in his great book of medical history around the time of the French Revolution, *The Birth of the Clinic: An archaeology of medical perception* (1973). Here he notes the transformation and opening up of the general table of medical knowledge in the second half of the eighteenth century: 'the treatises of the eighteenth century, institutions, aphorisms, nosologies enclosed medical knowledge within a defined space: the table drawn up may not have been complete in every detail, and may have contained gaps here and there owing to ignorance, but in its general form it was exhaustive and closed. It was now replaced by open, infinitely extendable tables' (Foucault 1973, p. 28).

This proliferation signalled the end of the primacy of the classificatory principle, and the eruption of a new curiosity about underlying causes, associations and generative principles of disease. The intensification of effort into elucidating medical knowledge produced not a filling-in of the general table, nor an extension of the table, but a pluralisation of medical knowledges, new disciplines and specialisations which subsequently ramified into the contemporary structures of medical science and medical practice.

The generative principle in these new knowledges was the understanding of the disease in a dynamic sense: of how the disease produced its effects; of the disease as a genetic principle. This was the initial possibility of the new therapeutics of medical intervention, aimed at the genetic principle of the disease itself, and designed to thwart its expression. It is in relation to this episteme of medicine that Foucault describes the development of the medical gaze within the teaching hospital. *The Birth of the Clinic* shows how the attention of physicians was turned to the internal organs of the body in all their gory detail: their sparkling membranes, intricate architecture, and contribution to life, as well as their suppurating inflammations, necrotic progressions and contribution to death.

Foucault has described in a programmatic way the institutional correlates of these developments in his short article 'The Politics of Health in the Eighteenth Century' (1980). Here he tells of the displacement of health services from the social assistance programs which was made possible by an analysis of idleness. Hospitals, previously organised as incarcereal institutions for the indigent, the mad or the biologically dangerous, emerged as 'the basis and sometimes the condition, for a more-or-less complex therapeutic approach. The Middlesex Hospital, intended for the treatment of smallpox and the practice of vaccination, was opened in London in 1745, the London Fever Hospital dates from 1802, and the Royal Ophthalmic Hospital from 1804. The first maternity hospital was opened in London 1749. In Paris the Enfants Malades was founded in 1802' (1980, p. 181).

The hospital system in the nineteenth century became organised around the organs: eye hospitals; ear, nose and throat hospitals; and general hospitals with wards devoted to the kidney, the heart, the bones, the brain, and so on. This was linked to an emerging division of labour within the health professions. A class- and gender-based division gave the various occupations: financier (often charitable), doctor, nurse, wardsman. But it was the organs which drove the division of each profession into its specialties: the neurosurgeon, the orthopaedic surgeon, the renal physician, the cardiologist, and so on. This list in the late twentieth century has become almost as long as the subheadings in an anatomy textbook.

THE ORIGINS OF PUBLIC HEALTH

The last section considered the development of hospital medicine in the nineteenth century, as it moved away from providing care for the indigent. The latter's numbers increased markedly during the nineteenth century—along with the growth of the world population as a whole—and became the subject of a growing governmental concern in the United Kingdom and elsewhere. This section considers the development of population health knowledges and public health practice within the biopolitics of that population expansion. During the time of the episteme of resemblance, the census developed as part of the tabular evaluation of the state. From the end of the eighteenth century, a genetic epistemology of populations emerged, along with a related practice of public health. In the second half of the nineteenth century, these developed specifically as technologies of communicable disease control, linked to the elaboration of the germ theory of disease.

While Foucault's investigations into the origins of biology and clinical medicine were central to his uncovering of what he called the modern episteme, his investigations into population were central to his development of ideas about governmentality. In the eighteenth century, he relates, 'the emergence of the health and physical well-being of the population in general as one of the essential objectives of political power' (Foucault 1980, pp. 169–70). He goes on to say: 'the project of a technology of population begins to be sketched: demographic estimates, the calculation of the pyramid of ages, different life expectations and levels of mortality, studies of the reciprocal relations of growth of wealth and the growth of population' (1980, p. 171).

The medical practitioner emerges with a central role in the new biopower regime:

> the doctor becomes the great adviser and expert, if not in the art of governing, at least in the art of observing, correcting and improving the social 'body' and maintaining it in a permanent state of health. And it is the doctor's function as hygienist rather than his prestige as a therapist that assures him this politically privileged position in the eighteenth century, prior to his accumulation of economic and social privileges in the nineteenth century (Foucault 1980, p. 177).

The contemporary history of public health is often commenced at this time. For example, the *Oxford Textbook of Public Health* (Holland et al.

1991) entry on the history of public health in the United Kingdom recounts: 'It was the report of three doctors in the aftermath of the 1832 Cholera epidemic that led the ubiquitous Victorian civil servant, Edwin Chadwick, to investigate "The sanitary conditions of the labouring poor". His famous report of 1842 emphasised the crucial link between dirt due to insanitary conditions and overcrowding and disease, and stressed the need for a central administrative structure to oversee health issues' (Lewis 1991, p. 25).

I shall return to this canonical history of the public health doctor shortly. A number of Foucault's admirers have also taken up the history of population science and public health in the nineteenth century, including Ian Hacking, a Cambridge-trained philosopher who now holds the Chair of History of Systems of Thought at the College de France, which was originally established for Foucault and which he held until his death in 1984. It is to Hacking's elaboration of the episteme of resemblance and its transformation into the modern genetic episteme in the field of population statistics that I now turn.

The great statistical tables of populations had their origins in censuses of Europe's colonies starting in 1548 in Peru and in the United States from 1776 when the census requirement was included in the US Articles of Confederation (Hacking 1990, Ch. 3). In 1700, the German philosopher, mathematician and statesman Leibniz had argued that:

> a Prussian state should be brought into existence, that the true measure of the state is its population, and that the state should have a central statistical office in order to know its power . . . He proposed a fifty-six category evaluation of state, which would include the number of people by sex, social status, the number of able-bodied men who might bear weapons, the number of marriageable women, the population density and age distribution, child mortality, life expectancy, distribution of diseases and causes of death (Hacking 1990, pp. 18–19).

Leibniz's great table of statistics (state-istics) would have provided a knowledge of the new state through the episteme of resemblance. Leibniz was a mathematician as well as a philosopher, an historian and a counsellor to nobility (Russell 1979). He developed the calculus (independently from Newton and with a clearer written exposition, aspects of which survive in present practice) as well as combinatorial analysis, the latter doing for categorical variables what the former does for continuous variables

(Bell 1953). At the origin of modern statistics, he gives us pause to remember that there are three common meanings of the term. First, statistics is the plural of statistic, a numerical fact: a count, ratio or proportion of something. Second, statistics is often thought of (especially by students) as a collection of mathematical techniques useful for the analysis of numerical facts, drawn from basic algebra, calculus, probability theory, matrix theory and so on. Third, statistics is a science or practice concerned with 'the classification, tabulation and study of numerical data' (Schwartz 1991, p. 1045). It refers to the ways of ordering things in the world into sets and series: a pragmatics of stating things in ways that can be analysed mathematically. As a practice, it is an evolving set of guidelines and instructions for determining unities or group membership, for counting and sampling, for creating arrays and for specifying allowable mathematical procedures, especially integrations towards summary statements which represent the world. As such, it has been developed and incorporated as a central component of the governmentality of modernity.

By 1784, Kant was noticing the internal regularities of the kinds of tables of statistics Leibniz had called for, postulating the existence of internal laws of nature which gave rise to these regularities:

> Deaths, births and marriages, considering how much they are separately dependant on the freedom of the human will, should seem to be subject to no law according to which any calculation could be made beforehand of their amount: and yet the yearly registers of these events in great countries prove that they go on with as much conformity to the laws of nature as the oscillations of the weather (Hacking 1990, p. 15).

In 1798, Malthus published *An Essay on the Principle of Population* (Malthus 1970), which discussed the propensity of populations to increase at a rate limited by the amount of food available—that is, at a rate determined by the check that lack of food places on the passions for sexual reproduction. Malthus's book has entered popular mythology, but the point I wish to note here is that it took population as its subject and sought to describe objectively a genetic principle (the 'principle of population') that provided an immanent motor for the historical development of populations.

By the mid-1820s, the English parliament's concerns for the governance of friendly societies led to the calculation of the quantum of sickness suffered by their members. The records of 73 societies covering 104 218 members, classified by age, by decade, with numbers of days off sick for a member, allowed a calculation to be made that around half a week a year of sickness was suffered by young men, rising to more than two weeks a year for those aged over 60 (Hacking 1990, p. 51).

This general quantum of sickness was then quickly elaborated upon. In the 1830s, William Farr in the office of the Registrar General of England developed a nosology—a taxonomy of diseases—and proposed a project of nosometry to measure the amount of these diseases in a population. Hacking reminds us that 'the very word [nosometry] reminds us that new classifications and new enumerations are inseparable' (Hacking 1990, p. 53).

Farr's nosology was the beginning of a proliferation of statistical collections that have maintained continuity through to today's International Classification of Diseases (10th edn) (WHO 1992): 'In 1893, a committee of the International Statistical Institute, chaired by Jacques Bertillon, produced a new classification based on Farr's principle which was known as the Bertillon or International Classification of Causes of Death' (NCCH 1997, section 2).

Conferences to revise the classification have been held every ten years or so ever since. From 1948 a classification of diseases was added, and the auspicing of the revision work fell to the World Health Organization, created in that year (NCCH 1997). Farr's work embodied the emergence in the nineteenth century of statistical tables which enabled the object of its enumerations—the population—to be interrogated for the genetic principles of disease which produced the regularities of the table.

The acme of theories about the internal principles of populations was Darwin's idea concerning the origin of species (i.e. populations of living things). He showed how the regular application of forces on a population arising from its environment acted through selection of the fittest—those best fitted in their environment—to produce evolutionary change in the population, and postulated that, given the right circumstances and sufficient time, one could expect to see the proliferation of several new species from one population. Darwin acknowledged the influence of Malthus's principle of population in the development of his theory (Flew 1970, p. 50), as did Wallace (Flew 1970, p. 51), and this accounts at least in part for the similarity of their two independently derived theories of evolution by natural selection.

Darwin's theory of evolution provided a convincing genetic principle for the origins of the various forms of life. Darwin's theory expressed the new episteme of generative principles in the epistemology of populations. This expression was echoed by embryology within the epistemology of animal biology and the germ theory of disease within medicine. Modern embryology investigates the genetic expression of germ cells into organs. The discipline in its contemporary form essentially dates from the establishment of the cell theory in 1839 by Schleiden and Schwann, and the realisation soon after that the human embryo develops from a single cell (Moore 1977, p. 9). The germ theory of disease shows how the genetic principle of organ function is corrupted and made pathological by an intersecting germ agent. The germ theory provided a scientific principle to underpin an emerging therapeutics of public health by explaining how personal hygiene and public sanitation measures stopped the transmission of disease. Perhaps the best way to illustrate this is to run through a brief history in the heroic style (notwithstanding the problems in this type of history) of various additions to the canon of clinical medicine in the nineteenth century.

A therapeutics based on interrupting the contagious spread of disease dates from Gordon's *Treatise on the Epidemic of Puerperal Fever in Aberdeen*, published in 1795: 'The basis of his argument is a table of 77 cases of puerperal fever. The table gives *inter alia* date and period of illness, age, residence, and by whom delivered' (Youngson 1979, p. 130). Out of the table, Gordon deduced that 'this disease seized such women only, as were visited, or delivered, by a practitioner, or taken care of by a nurse, who had previously attended patients affected with the disease . . . the nurses and physicians, who have attended patients affected with Puerperal fever, ought carefully to wash themselves, and to get their apparel properly fumigated, before it be put on again' (Youngson 1979, p. 130).

In the United Kingdom, techniques for the prevention of contagion made their way from the hospital to the town in 1854 (Jeffs 1994) when John Snow made a map of cholera cases in Soho (London) and tabulated the characteristics of the people affected. He deduced that water from the Broad Street pump was the cause of the outbreak. He convinced local authorities to remove the handle of the pump, and the outbreak quickly resolved.

Understanding of the link between germs and disease came a little later. Bretonneau identified a germ as the cause of the false membrane in the respiratory tract in diphtheria, and postulated that, in a similar way, each disease has a specific aetiology (Youngson 1979, p. 134). Pasteur disproved the theory of spontaneous generation in 1861 and invented pasteurisation (heat treatment of milk) in 1864; then Koch published the germ theory of disease in 1876 followed by his (and Jakob Henle's) postulates for establishing the microbiological aetiology of a disease in 1877 (Tortora et al. 1995, p. 9).

Let us now revert from an heroic history of scientific discovery to the social history of public health. Latour's history of the hygienists in France (Latour 1988, Ch. 1) delineates the alliance between hygienist knowledges and practices and the governing authorities of France during the 1850s and 1860s to cement the nineteenth century biopolitics regime. Somewhat paradoxically, acceptance of the germ theory by the early twentieth century led to a narrowing of medical influence on social reform:

> As a result of the germ theory, the twentieth century concept of dirt 'narrowed' so that it proved considerably cheaper to clean up . . . Once it was realized that dirt *per se* did not cause infectious disease, the broad mandate of public health to deal with all aspects of environmental sanitation and housing as a means of promoting cleanliness disappeared (Lewis 1991, p. 27).

In place of a broad interest in civic reform, public health practice developed its interests in communicable disease control towards the end of the nineteenth century and early in the twentieth century. This included the investigation and management of communicable disease outbreaks (e.g. cholera, typhoid, smallpox and bubonic plague) through the administration of various vaccines as they became available (smallpox, rabies) (in Australia, the Commonwealth government established the Commonwealth Serum Laboratories in 1916 to facilitate the development of vaccines: Gillespie 1991, p. 37), development of quarantine functions, and investigations into the communicable diseases of the tropical colonies of European countries.

PUBLIC HEALTH AND PUBLIC HOSPITALS

The development of communicable disease control within the practice of public health brought it closer to the more clinically oriented parts of the medical profession. Early in the twentieth century, it began to take up a deeper engagement with curative medicine and hospitals. The discipline of public health is now considered to have a twofold task: 'The prevention of disease and the promotion of health on the one hand, and the planning and evaluation of health services on the other' (Lewis 1991, p. 23). It is the latter task to which we now direct our attention.

In the United Kingdom, Chadwick's report of 1842 provoked the *Public Health Act* of 1848, which created the positions of medical officers of health (MOsH) in local government areas. By 1919, the chief medical officer of the Local Government Board (who oversaw the MOsH) argued 'for a new synthesis and integration in medicine, and in particular, a closer integration of preventive and curative medicine' (Lewis 1991, p. 28). In 1929, 'local authorities were permitted to take over the administration of the poor law hospitals, and many MOsH found themselves taking on the role of medical superintendent' (1991, p. 28). The establishment of the National Health Service (NHS) after the Second World War, however, separated the provision of public health advice and services from hospital administration. This was again reversed by the Thatcher reforms to the NHS, specifically the separation of purchaser from provider functions. This provided the opportunity for public health experts to develop roles in the purchasing authorities, working on the specification of volume, quality and location of hospital-based clinical services (UK Dept of Health 1989; Appleby 1992; Dugdale 1994).

In Australia, Gillespie has written an excellent history of the interaction between public health and clinical medicine for the period 1910–60 (Gillespie 1991; Dugdale 1992b). He describes the development of the National Hygiene Movement after the First World War, when 'medical colleagues returned to Australia filled with a desire to apply to the civil community the great lessons of successful medical control and prevention of disease which had been applied in the army' (Gillespie 1991, p. 31, quoting Cumpston, the founding director-general of the Commonwealth Health Department (1921–45)). The Commonwealth Department of Health was formed in 1921 in response to the Spanish flu epidemic of 1919, but faced constitutional impediments in the provision of health services.

Raphael Cilento, the most radical of the national hygienists (in a right-wing sense—he produced anti-democratic writings and had open sympathies with the Fascists in Italy and the Nazis in Germany) (Gillespie 1991, p. 35), moved from a position as Cumpston's deputy to become director-general of the Queensland Health Department in 1934 (1991, pp. 74–5). He planned to transform the department from a 'sleepy backwater concerned with the enforcement of sanitary regulations' (1991, p. 75) to a modern organisation administering all aspects of health service delivery, with a hierarchical model of authority extending down from his office 'through the large public hospitals to a decentralised system of district general hospitals and group clinics staffed by general practitioners and visiting specialists' (1991, p. 75). With the backing of Queensland's Labor government he was successful with the state's public hospitals, and overcame the ambivalence of the local medical profession about working under such arrangements by requiring all new graduates to serve a full year on salary in a public hospital before graduating. Although his plans to extend the organisation to private medical practice met with intractable resistance, he laid the foundations for free public hospital care and a tradition of centralised hospital planning in Queensland that has survived to the present day.

However, Queensland was the only state where this shotgun wedding between public health interests in the state health department and clinical medicine in the hospitals was brought about during the mid-twentieth century. At the Commonwealth level, during 1943 and 1944: 'Plans for a national health service based on salaried service and the integration of public and curative health services were discarded as the federal Labor government reduced its health scheme to a minor part of a wider pro-gramme of social security cash benefits' (Gillespie 1991, p. 131).

Commonwealth interest in actually providing public hospital services resurfaced under the Whitlam Labor government of 1972–75, during the planning for Medibank. The main proponent was Whitlam himself, but the idea was dropped after sustained opposition from the chairman of the Hospitals and Health Services Commission, Dr Sid Sax (Scotton and MacDonald 1993, p. 155). Instead, Sax was commissioned to undertake an inquiry into Australia's hospital system (Sax 1974). This report underpinned the various hospital funding agreements between the Commonwealth and several states which formed part of the Medibank system (for an account of these agreements, see Scotton and MacDonald 1993, Ch. 9).

FUNDING FORMULAS FOR PUBLIC HOSPITALS

Until the end of the 1970s public hospitals were traditionally funded—like most public sector agencies—on a line item basis. Their annual budget consisted of a large table with lines of expenditure listed down the left and columns of associated dollars. Lines corresponded to expenditure, not to function, and certainly not to population health needs.

In the 1980s, there was a move to global hospital funding. This was part of the new public sector managerialism associated with reviews by Coombs (1976) and Wilenski (1982) (Wilenski was a medical practitioner whose early understanding of institutions would have been formed in the hospital), and in the health system by Sax (1974) and then by Jamison (1980) during the dismantling of Medibank under the Fraser Liberal government (1975–83) (see Wooldridge 1991, Ch. 8, for a commentary on the Jamison inquiry).

The move to global funding was, of course, not the end of the budget table—merely the beginning of a proliferation of new ones. Inside the hospital, budgets began to reflect the functional divisions of professional practice based on the organ systems. There has been a shift in the organisation of labour within hospitals away from occupationally based divisions (medicine, nursing, allied health and ancillary) towards organ-centred divisions (cardiovascular, renal, reproductive, neurosciences). Frequently, each of these organ-based divisions has its own budget, and some are beginning to operate as enterprises within themselves (see Braithwaite 1993a, 1993b). This new organ-based regime of where the global budget goes is still emerging in Australia. Some hospitals have complex matrix management structures which reflect the transition. These matrixes locate each unit in the hospital in relation to the old regime of occupational divisions and the new regime of organ systems, and attempt to maintain dual accountability.

On the other side of the global budget—that is, where the budget comes from—the annual budget cycle bunfight has become systematised into formulas which divide the available health service funding. The traditional process of hospitals fighting over their own slice of funding was highly political, involving sensational media. Since the 1990s in Australia, within the public sector much of the struggle has been over the health service funding formula: the design of the pattern for cutting the cake as well as the size of the cake.

The New South Wales Resource Distribution Formula (RDF), introduced in the early 1990s, superseded the Resource Allocation Formula that provided indicative funding shares. The formula now carries much of the work of governing the New South Wales health system. The RDF provided the actual funding share of over $4 billion per annum according to six main components to the fifteen area health services. By 2005, the RDF had evolved to include nine major components (NSW Health 2005) and grown to distribute over $7 billion each year to the reorganised eight area health services. The purpose of the funds distributed by the RDF is to provide health services for the population within each area, whether provided by that area or by another area. The six main terms or components of the initial RDF were:

- population health services;
- non-inpatient services (dental; primary and community-based services; outpatients; and emergency department services);
- acute inpatient services;
- mental health services;
- rehabilitation and extended care; and
- teaching and research.

Needs-based equity in resource allocation remains the guiding principle in the RDF. Factors that are used to weight the share of the various programs each area gets include the following:

- population share (age/sex rated);
- need, as defined by standardised mortality ratios and measures of socioeconomic status and rurality;
- Aboriginality and homelessness;
- private hospital flows;
- private/public mix;
- severity (NSW Health 1996c, pp. 4–5).

The last three factors provide incentives within the formula to increase public hospital treatment within areas, and to treat more severe patients within areas. All of the components provide incentives to increase volumes of services provided (with the exception of population health services). In addition, three incentive pools were established, distributed according to area activity in line with pool objectives. Incentive funds have been provided for:

- waiting time reduction;
- emergency services; and
- outcome improvement.

The initial RDF regime required each area to develop the following documents:

- an acute care flow plan;
- flow impact statement;
- area service plan; and
- health improvement plan.

These provided the basis for areas to contract internally with their own service agencies and externally with other areas for the provision of services. These contracts specified price and volume of services in terms of diagnosis-related groups (DRGs). I return to the New South Wales RDF case study in the final chapter, to show how the enunciation of the formula was related to opportunities for policy activism at the statewide level. In this chapter, I am more concerned with the impact of the RDF at the hospital level.

The New South Wales health system is one of the largest in the world, and provides comprehensive hospital and community health services to around 5 million people. The RDF regime is complex and its implementation involved a ten-year process. The early evidence was that doctors hated it: when it was first introduced, market research by the Institute for Social Research showed that only 8 per cent had confidence in decisions made by health system management. Like an ocean liner being brought around (a metaphor Appleby (1992) used in describing Thatcher's reforms to the National Health Service), perceptible changes in response to formula drivers occurred slowly, but have now been built into the fabric of the health system.

The organ-based divisions within hospitals, where these have emerged, are faced with the task of operating within a population needs-based planning regime. Full clinical freedom is retained within these units, but it is a market-like freedom: to be poorer or richer; to resist change and suffer or seize opportunities and prosper. The clinician managers in charge of these divisions, those old organ grinders, are being taught the population health improvement march. Their scientific interests are developing to encompass population health matters and techniques, in addition to their traditional bench science. The population health relevance of the clinical activities of these new divisions is being articulated—sometimes forcefully, often in the context of the budget cycle.

On the other side of the fence, public health units have been established in all areas, where they are involved deeply in the planning and budget process. Traditionally antagonistic to—and marginalised from—hospital-based clinical medicine, they are now assisting in articulating the population health relevance of clinical units. Their entrée into this world has not just been because of their closeness to the budget process. It is also based on their knowledge of epidemiological trial design and biostatistical analysis—two key tools in contemporary clinical research. The clinical/population health alliances developing within area health services are a key factor in the reestablishment of medical hegemony within the new regime. As Foucault reminds us, ' "private" and "socialised" medicine, in their reciprocal support and opposition, both derive from a common global strategy' (1980, p. 161).

Funding formulas as a financing technology are linked to the population sciences. The formulas rely on the enumeration of the population, its breakdown by geography, age and sex, its morbidity and mortality, and its propensity to use health services. In this assemblage, the state seeks legitimacy in the provision of health services through establishing a relationship with the population sciences. Because funds are provided at the population level, population measures of service use and the benefits resulting from services (health outcomes) are desirable for building incentives for improved performance into the structure of the formula. Population-based illness prevention and health promotion also come into sharp focus as potentially effective and efficient ways to provide services.

We can recognise this as the funding formula/population sciences assemblage of the health system discussed in Chapter 3. An increasing proportion of the health sector is being organised along these lines, and the importance of the old health insurance/clinical sciences assemblage is waning. This transformation from the old to the new assemblage in the governmentality of health is particularly influential in relation to changes occurring in the institutional design of the health system, and to changes in the way medicine is practised, including the introduction of new clinical technologies.

The principal form of aggregation of health care providers in this assemblage is in health services, funded as health care provider agencies by the formulas. The principal form of aggregation of health care recipients is as populations with both health care needs and influence on the election of governments. Strong relationships between these two forms of aggregation are developing, and we can perhaps term this the pastoralisation of health care services. It is within this relationship that we see the emergence of profound implications for knowledge produced by the population sciences in the exercise of power throughout the health system.

Within this assemblage, funding formulas have emerged as the principal distributive mechanism for funding public sector health services. Formulas have developed as a specific technology that deploys a certain type of rationality developed in processes of recurrent budgeting. They are now used to fund the Commonwealth–State Medicare Agreements, as well as hospital services in most states, and in the Commonwealth government's Practice Incentives Program for general practices.

Funding formulas carry the governmentality of health by producing relationships between science, services and finances. In this way, they constitute the contemporary assemblage of the health system. Like all governmental statements, they operate between the articulable and the visible: between articulated governmental policy and visible health services. As policy statements, funding formulas deploy population and service activity data to reflexively affect the delivery of services and the health characteristics of the population. The formulas distribute funds from health department budgets for specified purposes to service delivery agencies as determined by the institutional design of the health system— state governments, area health services, hospitals, general practices, and so on. The formulas are an integrative mathematical function which typically combines population, service delivery and financial data with an incentive structure to encourage desired service characteristics.

This loop constitutes population health as a field of governmental activity that was not previously possible, and has wrought a contemporary alchemy in the politics of health that places the public health discipline at centre stage. Now, many of the most important arguments over resource allocation are couched in the terms of the formulas: the institutional design; the population base; adjustments for mortality, service use and efficiency; and the incentive structure in determining who gets how much to do what. These terms have themselves largely been derived from public health and related disciplines, including public policy and health economics.

The enunciation of funding formulas occurs within a network of governmental statements: they may be determined as necessary by an Act of parliament; their form may be specified in an agreement between agencies; their incentive structure may need to reflect previously elaborated policy objectives. This enunciation then orchestrates a series of conjunctions between surveillance data from many sources in the calculation of actual resource allocations.

The transition in the health field to the new funding formula/ population sciences assemblage has implications for the tactics of health politics, for the form of health services, for the discipline of public health and population sciences, and for both patients and health policy activists. In health politics, we can expect to see the application of funding formulas to new areas of health resource allocation. Each time this occurs, we need to be alive to the possibilities for pursuing population health approaches that this opens up and the tactical advantages it can confer.

The implementation of the new assemblage presents real opportunities to reorganise and coordinate health services to achieve the required population focus. The changes in the forms and structures of health services resulting from the shift to the funding formula/population sciences diagram presents opportunities for public health professional bodies such as the Public Health Association and the Australasian Faculty of Public Health Medicine to strengthen their interest and leadership in the organisation and administration of health services, where they may provide a rallying point for an expansion of health service resources against the secular trend of economic rationalism and cost constraint in public welfare services.

The research agenda for public health must itself respond to the new assemblage. Because of the traditional close relationship the specialty of public health has with the population sciences, the public health disciplines have found themselves at centre stage in the health funding policy arena. This newfound importance goes beyond the wildest dreams of the new public health revival of the 1980s. These disciplines are caught in the spotlight, blinking, unsure of their role in influencing the health system and with a manifestly inadequate knowledge base to work from. The challenge is to further develop knowledges relating health services to population outcomes, and to identify ways of facilitating these links through innovations in the incentive structure of health service funding formulas. Activity in these areas accounts for some of the more innovative research currently being carried out in public health. One line of this research program is concerned with the improvement of health outcomes through adjustments to clinical practice and service development (e.g. Ellwood 1988; NSW Health Department 1991a, 1992; and the research program of the Menzies

Centre for Health Policy and Practice). This adopts a line of public sector rationalisation drawing on strategic management approaches (for a discussion of this, see Offe 1984, p. 111). Lately, this has converged with a research program on evidence-based medicine, which has similar objectives but is bound up with a more distributed, collegial style of practice. An underlying program of research into medical practice variation (Andersen and Mooney 1990) is related to the quality movement approach developed in US and Japanese industry during the 1960s, which was taken up by the health sector in the 1980s (Prevost et al. 1992; Shaw et al. 1991) (see Chapter 7).

The implications for patients of the new assemblage are complex. Funding formulas like the Australian Health Care Agreements and the New South Wales RDF do not require an active subject position to be taken by patients: patient involvement is as part of a population, as a collection of bodies to be enumerated and located. These formulas engage the medical profession in a struggle over institutional structure and control, especially with respect to the hospital. This has profound implications for medical training, research and career development (the specifiers of the doctor's subject position). The effects on styles of patient care and the operation of the doctor–patient relationship are far more subtle and not so direct. On this interpretation, funding formulas enable the positive implementation of strategies of increasing equity without adversely affecting the private relationship of the patient with their doctor—an important property of an administrative technology in a society touched by a 'radical disenchantment with the state' (Papadakis and Taylor-Gooby 1987).

Health service funding formulas express the episteme of modernity. They contain internal genetic principles which generate funding shares. This approach represents a profound transformation of the historical tabular form of hospital financing. But there is a marked difference from the process which Foucault described at the end of the Classical age: he characterised the genetic principle as an element in the construction of knowledge. Here we see it appear as a principle in the expression of state power—as an administrative tool.

Funding formulas carry a number of funding principles. Like many administrative technologies, they perform policy work on a number of different fronts. Their reliance on population needs analysis is directed towards achieving allocative efficiency; their reliance on case mix analysis is directed towards achieving throughput efficiency; the outcomes incentives pool is directed towards achieving effectiveness. These policy principles are the genetic code in the funding formulas. Unlike the genetic principles of organ function discovered by the biologists, these administrative principles were *chosen* for insertion into the funding formula. When doctors elaborated a therapeutic vision through the creation and manipulation of genetic principles in the human organism, they were accused of playing God. With the development of administrative technologies capable of carrying a diverse array of principles of government, we are witnessing a mode of government in which the formula-wielding system administrator has replaced the pork-barrelling sovereign god king.

Yet already the funding formula technology is proving inadequate for the demands of the new public health assemblage of the health system. There is a Holy Grail that would ensure that funding formulas live on forever within the assemblage. This is the development of health outcome drivers—incentives that operate within the formula to improve the health outcomes of services and the health of the population. Such drivers have proved elusive. The problem is that the marginal effect of such drivers is to gradually give a population a greater share of available resources as its health improves. This contradicts the equity orientation of the entire funding formula approach. My guess is that stable, long-term drivers within formulas can only be directed towards improving efficiency, and that drivers for improved effectiveness and health outcomes need to be chopped and changed as the evidence of what needs to be done comes to hand. This will create difficulties because change to an established formula will always face considerable resistance. But perhaps I am wrong: perhaps the cleverness of formula technicians will translate into a successful development of stable health outcomes drivers. Time will tell.

This chapter has taken a long-wave analysis of the interaction between the clinical medicine and the public health discourses. It began by showing how both rest on elaborations of knowledge conducted within the modern episteme of genetic principles, and concluded by examining the latest juxtaposition of the two discourses in the contemporary public hospital setting, including a discussion of funding formulas. Such a long-term historical analysis is useful because of the historical stability of the hospital system and the longevity of discursive formations within hospitals. For the policy analyst, it can counterbalance the obsession with the power struggles of the day, which often determine debate.

6.

THE MAKING OF MEDICARE

As a teenager in the 1970s, I grew up in a large, politically engaged family in the suburban plains of Adelaide. The politics was pretty interesting, with conscription being abolished, Vietnamese refugees arriving, a premier who championed the arts, a prime minister who got sacked and a new national health scheme every year or so right through until the mid-1980s. For people entering the world of health policy in the last two decades, it must have been hard to imagine the volatility of health policy in the period 1972–85. For contemporary health economists, the logic of ending universal health coverage in September 1981, leaving around 2 million Australians without health insurance, must be almost unfathomable.

Against this backdrop, the introduction of the Hawke Labor government's Medicare health policy was an event of major social and political importance. The making of Medicare involved the nationalisation of medical insurance, the opening of public hospitals to provide free comprehensive treatment to anyone who needed it, extensive regulation of private health insurance, and a major expansion in the clinical freedom of health professionals. These major structural elements remain largely in place today.

Australia's public hospital networks and Commonwealth Medical Benefits Scheme are the mainstays of the Commonwealth government's Medicare policy. With the intensification of governments' interest in health as they became involved in financing health care, the electoral politics of health were elaborated in more detail. The physicians' populations were recognised as the politicians' electorates, and health care was elevated to a hip pocket issue. The chapter concludes by considering the impact of Medicare on clinical freedom and locates this within a line of argument in political philosophy concerning the administration of freedom by the state.

THE MICROECONOMICS OF MAKING MEDICARE

After the Second World War, attempts by the Commonwealth Labor government to create a national health service similar to that in the United Kingdom were frustrated by political opposition and constitutional problems of federation, but resulted in the establishment of the Pharmaceutical Benefits Scheme in the late 1940s. Subsequently, the Menzies government established the Medical Benefits Scheme in the mid-1950s. As part of the establishment of Medibank, insurance for medical services was nationalised by the Whitlam government in 1975. The budget legislation associated with this eventually precipitated Whitlam's dismissal by the Governor-General in November that year. The Fraser government had substantially dismantled Medibank by 1981; however, the Hawke government once more nationalised insurance for medical services in 1983 as part of the establishment of Medicare. This development towards state financing of health care—which occurred throughout the OECD in the second half of the twentieth century—has been motivated by the increasing efficacy of expert medical interventions and the increasing difficulty consumers have in assessing their value.

A summary understanding of Medicare is necessary to follow the discussion in this chapter. At the most fundamental level, Medicare can be summarised as three main things:

- First, Medicare is the name of a policy commitment to a national health system which features universal access to comprehensive services. At the point of service delivery, these are either free or incur only a small charge to the patient. At every Australian election since 1983 (and some would argue since 1973), this policy has received an electoral mandate.
- Second, Medicare entailed the definition of a set of benefits—Medicare benefits—to be paid by the government to patients who received medical services from doctors outside of public hospitals. Corresponding to this set of benefits is a package of regulations concerning private health insurance.

- Third, Medicare involves a set of contracts—the Australian Health Care Agreements (AHCAs)—which provide the states with money for their hospital systems and define the states' responsibilities in contributing to the national plan of universal comprehensive access to services. The state responsibilities relate largely to public hospital services, but also include some community-based services.

The Australian Health Care Agreements are a series of eight agreements between the Commonwealth government and each state and territory government (I use the term 'states' to denote all states, the Australian Capital Territory and the Northern Territory). The agreements commit the Commonwealth government to providing specific-purpose grants to the states (under section 96 of the Constitution) for the purpose of providing public hospital services, and the states to providing comprehensive public hospital services with universal access to the public based on medical need. The agreements recognise that the states will need to provide a similar level of funds from other sources to meet this commitment. The agreements cover a five-year period, the agreements at the time of writing being from 2003 to 2008. There have been three previous sets of agreements covering 1988 to 1993, 1993 to 1998 (called the Commonwealth State Medicare Agreements (CSMA)) and 1998 to 2003. The period to 1988 from the introduction of Medicare in February 1984 was covered by a number of slightly disparate agreements reflecting the transition from the various pre-Medicare funding arrangements in force in different states.

The 2003–08 agreement distributed approximately $42 billion in Commonwealth funds, or $8.4 billion per annum, between the states according to a formula (the AHCA formula) specified in the agreements. The AHCAs and the AHCA formula can be analysed as a series of statements with a set of referents. The AHCA relates to a series of objects, subjects, concepts and strategies that constitute the field of referents within which it is situated.

The main objects which the AHCAs reference are the financial resources provided by the Commonwealth government and the health services provided by the state governments. The main subject positions to be taken with reference to the AHCAs are the various institutions of the Commonwealth and state governments. Others, such as taxpayers and private health insurance companies, are also referred to.

The conceptual field within which the AHCAs are enunciated is the field of health policy statements (the AHCAs make many references to other statements of health policy, particularly matters discussed at the Australian Health Ministers Council), other government statements, and other statements forming the discourse on health—largely dominated by the medical profession.

The strategic field of the AHCAs can broadly be termed the field of health politics, including the articulation of health matters with the politics of the Commonwealth and state governments, especially with regard to financial appropriations. The major formative events of the strategic field were the emergence of the Commonwealth government as by far the largest purchaser in the health service market; the alignment of medical, private health insurance and private hospital lobbies against Commonwealth and state governments (especially New South Wales) in the doctors' strike in 1984–85 (see Daniel 1990); and the pitting of these three lobbies against each other with the development of the private health insurance reforms by the Commonwealth in the latter half of the 1990s.

The remainder of this case study on the making of Medicare focuses on the major shifts in the financing of health services. It examines governmental action to transform the health system from one that relied largely on private health insurance to the Medicare system that relies largely on public sector funding. Market-based distributional mechanisms are replaced by a formula-based distribution mechanism. Market incentives—which do not operate in the health system according to the traditional market model—are replaced by the financial incentives determined by the formula, both explicit in the operation of the bonus pools (schedules D and E of the 2003–08 AHCA), and implicit with regard to cost-shifting between various health service programs.

The key practical question in the historical analysis of this transformation is how the resources for the introduction of Medicare were brought together. This section tells the story of the making of the pie that would be distributed by the CSMA formula in the refinancing of the health system. It commences by examining trends in current health expenditure before looking at the way the base for the CSMA was determined.

Health service funding formulae can in general be regarded as public sector funding mechanisms. This section considers the transfer of health financing into the public sector. This transfer provides the context in which the size of the pie that the AHCA funding formula distributes is determined.

In 2003–04, total expenditure on health was estimated to be $78.6 billion a year, or 9.7 per cent of GDP. Some $26.4 billion of this was spent on acute hospital services. Total government expenditure on health was $53.2 billion, of which $35.4 billion was Commonwealth government expenditure (AIHW 2006, p. 436). This puts into context the $8.4 billion the Commonwealth government distributes annually through the AHCA formula, mainly for acute public hospital services.

Health expenditure as a share of GDP was 6.4 per cent in 1970–71, rising to 7.6 per cent in 1975–76, coinciding with the introduction of Medibank. It then remained stable right through the 1980s and the introduction of Medicare until the recession of 1990–91, with health expenditure growing at between 3 and 4 per cent a year, similar to overall GDP growth but without the cyclical variation of the latter (see Table 6.1).

Table 6.1 Health expenditure as a share of GDP

Health expenditure		Health expenditure	
Year	as % GDP	Year	as % GDP
1970–71	6.4	1993–94	8.3
1975–76	7.6	1994–95	8.3
1983–84	7.7	1995–96	8.4
1984–85	7.7	1996–97	8.6
1985–86	7.7	1997–98	8.6
1986–87	8.0	1998–99	8.7
1987–88	7.8	1999–00	8.9
1988–89	7.7	2000–01	9.2
1989–90	7.8	2001–02	9.4
1990–91	8.2	2002–03	9.6
1991–92	8.4	2003–04	9.7
1992–93	8.5		

Sources: AIHW 1994, p. 281; AIHW 2006, p. 290.

The trend in health expenditure is that it increases as a percentage of GDP as GDP itself increases. In other words, the wealthier a country becomes the more it spends on health. As Australia has become wealthier over the last few decades, it has spent an extra 1 per cent of GDP on health care each decade.

If we accept this as the long-term trend, the introduction of Medicare in the mid-1970s increased health expenditure as a percentage of GDP relative to the trend, after which it remained fairly flat through the introduction of Medicare, eventually falling below the trend through until 1990. During the national recession of 1990–91 (when GDP actually fell), health expenditure jumped back up to the long-term trend line and has continued its gradual increase since.

Against this background of stable overall health expenditure from 1975 to 1990, the introduction of Medicare in 1983–84 occurred with a shift of financing share from the private sector to the Commonwealth government. In 1982–83, the Commonwealth government contributed 33.7 per cent of total health expenditure, and the private sector contributed 39.8 per cent. By 1984–85, the Commonwealth's contribution had risen to 45.6 per cent and the private sector's contribution had declined to 28.9 per cent (AIHW 1994).

How did this come about? The private sector contribution declined because of a reduction in private health insurance coverage. First, the Commonwealth government passed a law (the Commonwealth *Health Insurance Act 1983*) making it illegal to offer insurance for fees charged by medical practitioners, thus reducing the scope of the private insurance products available. Second, the provision of universal access to comprehensive, free hospital services as part of the Medicare program resulted in many people dropping their private health insurance, which by then mainly covered only hospital fees, not doctors' fees. The proportion of the population with private health insurance covering acute hospital care dropped from 61.5 per cent in December 1983 to 47.9 per cent in December 1984 (AIHW 1994, p. 288). Third, the Commonwealth reduced its direct cash subsidy to the health insurance industry reinsurance pool (a trust fund operated by the Commonwealth, in which all private health insurance operators were obliged to participate by the *Private Health Insurance Act*) from $100 million in 1983–84 to $20 million in 1984–85 (CDH 1984, pp. 101–2).

Parallel to this, the increase in Commonwealth government contribution to health expenditure occurred in two main programs. First, the program of medical benefits for low income earners operated by the Commonwealth Department of Health since the mid-1980s was expanded to cover the whole population. Medical benefits paid by the Commonwealth increased from $917 million in 1982–83 to $1364 million in 1983–84 (CDH 1984, p. 202). It had risen to $2887 million by 1986–87 (AIHW 1994, p. 292) and to

$10.93 billion by 2005–06 (Medicare Australia 2006, p. 90). (By way of comparison, if Commonwealth outlays on medical benefits had increased by inflation alone, according to the specific price deflators used by the AIHW (AIHW 1994, p. 279), $917 million in 1982–83 would have grown to $978 million in 1983–84 and to $1110 million in 1986–87.)

Medicare benefits reimburse patients for the medical services they receive. It remains up to the patient to pay the doctor for their services. Responsibility for administering the benefits scheme was transferred from the Commonwealth Health Department to the Health Insurance Commission (HIC) (now Medicare Australia), which at that time operated Medibank Private, the government's own private health insurance company, established in 1976. The HIC then expanded its network of Medibank shopfronts, renamed Medicare offices, which provided the interface with the public in relation to this program.

Moving on to hospital outlays, the Commonwealth increased its payments to the states by $188 million in 1983–84 and $704 million in 1984–85 to reimburse them for agreeing to implement the Medicare policy (agreed to by all states and the Northern Territory at the Premiers' Conference of June 1983), for allowing everyone free access to the public hospitals the states operated, and to make up for the expected shortfall in revenue paid by private health insurance funds to public hospitals (CDH 1984, pp. 101–2).

The key determinants of the amount of money distributed by the Commonwealth government to state governments to fund the Medicare agreements can be summarised as follows:

- the amounts paid by the Commonwealth to state governments for hospital services prior to Medicare (in block grants to New South Wales, Queensland, Victoria and Western Australia since the ending of hospital cost-sharing arrangements between the Commonwealth and those states after 1981; and through continuing hospital cost-sharing arrangements with South Australia and Tasmania);
- the constriction of private health insurance financing of health services by: 1) reducing the propensity of the population to take out private health insurance by guaranteeing free access to universal health services in public hospitals; 2) reducing government contributions to the reinsurance pool by $80 million; and 3) the restriction to $80 per day of the amount for hospital services that public

hospitals could charge private patients in shared wards (funded by 'Basic Hospital Cover'), around one-third of the comparable charge made by private hospitals;
- the complementary increase in demand for publicly funded public hospital services from people who had previously held private health insurance, and the additional increase in demand from people who were previously uninsured;
- taking these factors into account, the Commonwealth government's calculation of the amount it needed to pay to the states to implement the policy, the state governments' calculation of the amounts they would need to implement the policy, and the outcome of bargaining between the Commonwealth and state governments over these amounts.

This amount formed the historical basis for the size of the pie to be distributed in later years by the AHCA funding formula. It is linked directly to the history of hospital funding in Australia and the architecture of the reforms to the health system by which Medicare was implemented.

The next major changes to the Medicare system occurred in 1988. A number of relatively minor technical changes—designed to make the implementation of the community rating principle fairer—were made to private health insurance reinsurance arrangements, and the Commonwealth ceased its annual $20 million contribution to the pool (Commonwealth DCSH 1989b, p. 72). At the 1988 Premiers' Conference, all state governments agreed to new arrangements for funding public hospitals under Medicare. The new Commonwealth–State Medicare Agreements (since renamed the Australian Health Care Agreements) were for five years (July 1988 to June 1993) and funding arrangements were more formularised. The total amount to be distributed included the following:

- a base grant from the Commonwealth of $3043 million per annum, replacing all previous Commonwealth grants to the states for the specific purpose of funding public hospitals, the amount to be increased annually to take account of price and wage movements, the growth of the population and the ageing of the population; and
- an incentives package consisting of $41 million per annum of Commonwealth money to encourage reduction in length of hospital stay, the introduction of case mix-based hospital management and funding systems to fund the hospital-based treatment of people with AIDS.

Funds were to be distributed by a formula that took into account the following:

- state population numbers;
- administrative costs, with lower costs per episode of care expected of larger states;
- the age and sex makeup of those populations, allowing for the varying hospital utilisation of different age/sex cohorts;
- levels of public patient utilisation of public hospitals in each state;
- levels of public hospital income from private patients' Medicare benefits paid by the HIC, applied as a cutoff above which penalties applied;
- numbers of AIDS patients being treated in each state (Commonwealth DCSH 1989b, pp. 74–5; Australian Government Solicitor 1993).

The next agreement covered the period July 1993 to June 1998. It was preceded by the Commonwealth passing the *Medicare Agreements Act 1992* 'to confirm the Medicare Principles of choice, universality and equity in service provision and the Medicare Commitments' (Commonwealth DHHLG&CS 1993, p. 46).

In the 1993–98 agreements, the previous agreements' base grant, indexed as specified in that agreement, now totalled $20 billion in hospital funding grants at 1992 prices over the five years. The Commonwealth supplemented this with an additional $1.59 billion at 1992 prices for the five years of the new agreement. This arrested a decline in the Commonwealth's share of public hospital funding that had occurred over the previous decade (Macklin 1991, p. 28).

Penalty clauses in the previous agreements, relating to penalties if private patient utilisation levels reached a certain cutoff, had proved unenforceable because data on which to base such decisions were not routinely collected by the Commonwealth. These clauses were replaced by a bonus pool arrangement which provided an incentive to increase the proportion of public patients treated (Australian Government Solicitor 1993, Schedule D). The new agreements also included data-submission procedures (1993, Schedule J).

So far, we have been examining the transformations of health financing from the perspective of health policy, specifically the implementation of the Medicare policy. The focus has been on changes to the flow of money:

the partial, forced replacement of private sector health insurance finance flows with public sector flows, and an overall increase in total flows to fund health care for people not previously receiving it under the previous financing regime. The next section broadens the analysis to examine the expansion of public sector health expenditure in the context of the Commonwealth government's taxation and fiscal policy settings.

GOVERNING HEALTH INSURANCE IN THE MEDICARE ERA

I have shown above how the transfer of financing from private health insurance to public sector financing systems was effected. Closely related to this transfer were two factors which fundamentally changed the nature of the health insurance market.

First, changes to the *Health Insurance Act* which came into force in early 1984 limited the types of health insurance products that could be offered in Australia. 'Basic' hospital insurance covered public hospital services. 'Supplementary' hospital insurance covered private hospital services, and could only be offered as a supplement to basic cover. 'Ancillary' insurance covered non-hospital, non-medical services such as allied health care (dentistry, physiotherapy, etc.) and therapeutic goods (spectacles, wheelchairs, etc.) that were and continue to be available in the public system only on a strictly means-tested basis.

Second, Medicare provided comprehensive health insurance cover for the whole population, thus drastically altering the nature of the choice faced by people considering purchasing health insurance. Concerning hospital-based services, instead of a choice between paying as they went or insuring for these costs, people now faced a choice between relying on the free public system or insuring themselves so they could be private patients in the public system (with the benefit of choice of doctor and perhaps a single room if one were available) or going to a private hospital.

The effect of these changes to the health insurance market in the first decade of Medicare can be summarised as follows.

The proportion of the population covered by private insurance for hospital services dropped sharply at the introduction of Medicare, and continued to fall more slowly over the next decade:

The proportion of the population holding private hospital insurance ['basic' cover] has fallen from about 68% in 1982 (prior to the introduction of Medicare), to 50.0% in June 1984 and 38.4% in December 1993. The fall was rapid around the introduction of Medicare, but then slowed to 0.8 percentage points per year from June 1984 to June 1989 . . . From June 1989 to December 1993 the rate of decrease for Australia remained fairly steady at 1.6% per year (AIHW 1994, pp. 137–8).

The proportion of private health insurance policy-holders with supplementary insurance, and thus access to private hospitals, increased from 46.8 per cent at the end of 1983 to 62.6 per cent at the end of 1984, and to 91.9 per cent by 1993 (calculated from data presented in AIHW 1994, p. 288).

The mix of people holding health insurance changed as the decade from 1984 progressed, with those taking out insurance becoming older, sicker and more likely to use health services. Premiums increased in line with this higher service use profile, and this price increase is likely to have caused the acceleration in the dropout rate from private health insurance during the 1990s (for a comprehensive review, see Industry Commission 1997). This in turn led to the introduction from 1997 of tax breaks for private health insurance and the introduction of lifetime cover discounts, which have seen the percentage of the population with private health insurance increase from a low of 30 per cent in December 1998 to 43 per cent in 2006 (Private Health Insurance Administration Council website, www.phiac.gov.au).

After a step down at the introduction of Medicare, private health insurance as a proportion of total health expenditure increased slightly between 1985 and 1994, as did the proportion of hospital admissions funded by private health insurance and the proportion of total hospital bed days that were funded by private health insurance. In 1994, private health insurance accounted for 11.2 per cent of the community's total expenditure on health (Industry Commission 1997, p. 21). This had fallen to 10.3 per cent by 2003–04, including tax rebates totalling 3.2 per cent of total health expenditure (AIHW 2006, p. 310).

The introduction of Medicare in the period 1983–85 posed specific problems for the governmentality of private health insurance, concerning its financial constriction, the delimitation of a range of products suitable for the altered health insurance market, and linking its operation to the new roles defined within Medicare for private and public hospitals. Politically, these changes reinforced the traditional alliance between the health insurance lobby, the medical specialists and the private hospitals. Together, these groups mounted a concerted, high-profile campaign against the new system, without succeeding in achieving fundamental changes.

After the introductory period, the issues in the governmentality of private health insurance changed. From 1985, the governmental problems of most concern were the continued viability of private health insurance and the maintenance of its contribution off the government budget to the health system, and ensuring appropriate linkages between private health insurance, private doctors, private hospitals, and the public hospital system.

Concerning linkages to the public system, the government adjusted the public health financing system to take private insurance financing into account, ensuring that public hospital resources were sufficient to match demand. Penalty clauses in the 1988–92 CSMA and the bonus pool in the 1993–98 AHCA formula were directed at adjusting state shares to account for different private insurance coverage in each state, and to discourage state governments from pushing people into private health insurance by reducing the quality or availability of public services compared with private services.

Concerning the linkages to private doctors and private hospitals, the area of most concern was the multiple bills people received for private care, itemised for many separate services, with the insurance benefit covering 100 per cent of some items and 85 per cent of others, with some covered 75 per cent by Medicare benefits with private insurance covering the remaining 25 per cent, and still other items not covered at all. Amendments were made to the *Private Health Insurance Act*, taking effect in 1995; these allowed a new product of combined medical and hospital cover where each episode of illness was treated as a single event, with a single bill (covering medical, hospital and diagnostic services, and pharmaceuticals) that was covered 100 per cent by the insurance benefit (for a listing of allowable private health insurance products, see Industry Commission 1997, p. 105).

It was hoped that new insurance products that could be developed under these regulations would be quite attractive in the transformed health insurance market of the Medicare era. Politically, these changes were supported by the private health insurance lobby and opposed by medical specialists (the AMA) and the private hospital lobby, on the grounds that they would transfer some effective control of private health sector operation to the insurers. Negotiation of 100 per cent cover arrangements between the funds, doctors and hospitals has been extremely slow.

Coincidentally, in the discussion period for these reforms (1992–95), when the traditional alliance between private health insurance, medical specialists and private hospitals broke up, the Liberal/National Coalition (in opposition from 1983) dropped its long-running opposition to Medicare and endorsed the key policy plank of universal coverage and the key administrative mechanism of bulk billing by doctors for benefits assigned to them by their patients. The 1995 reforms to the private health insurance regulations were passed with bipartisan support. The governmentality of private health insurance in the period 1985–95 was thus effective in stymying opposition to Medicare and politically stabilising the new assemblage of the health system. The Liberal/National Coalition won government at the federal election in March 1996 and continued to support Medicare in office. It introduced a number of changes to health financing arrangements, particularly tax incentives for private health insurance which, along with a loosening of community rating rules, have arrested or partially reversed the decline in private health insurance coverage rates, thus further stabilising Australia's overall mix of public and private health insurance arrangements.

The introduction of Medicare in 1983–84 and the attendant changes to private health insurance regulations left the private health insurance system in a state of disequilibrium. Specifically, the entire population became self-insured for all medical and hospital treatment. This led to a continuing drop in the number of people willing to pay for private health insurance until the private health insurance reforms of 1997–2000. The mix of people insured privately also changed as people with a higher need for health care stayed in, and the young and fit left more readily. Community risk rating— meaning that policies had to be offered to everyone at the same price, no matter what their age or risk profile—increased the difference in dropout rates according to need. Premiums drifted up. Remarkably, total money through private insurance increased steadily after the initial stepwise decline in 1984, as did bed days financed. This was assisted by a speculative private hospital bed investment boom in the late 1980s.

A second instability existed from 1984 to 1995 in the form of a lack of political consensus on the publicly insured medical service payment system of Medicare benefits. Gradually, however, public support waned for the

Liberal Party position of opposition to key elements of Medicare, both among patients and doctors. In 1995, the Liberal Party-led opposition came out in support of universal bulk billing, thus stabilising the political ground and regulatory framework of this major arm of the health financing system.

The Commonwealth–State Medicare Agreements received little attention on the parliamentary political stage. It was the health care delivery end of this financing system—the public hospitals—that received attention, spectacularly in the form of industrial disputes between specialist doctors, public hospitals and Labor governments, both state and federal. The 1988 agreement was reached with little fanfare in the period immediately after an election (October 1987). The financing end gained some publicity in the 1993 agreement because agreement occurred immediately before the federal election in March 1993. The 1998 and 2003 agreements received some press coverage, but did not make much impact on the political landscape at this time.

I would like now to give an example of the tactics of government associated with the shift to formula-based resource allocation. The AHCAs are an instrument used to implement the Medicare policy as articulated by the Commonwealth government. They are agreements precisely about the formula for calculating Commonwealth funding to the states and the specific services that must be seen to be provided with these funds.

The 1988 Agreement specified a grant to be paid to each state, calculated on the basis of standardised population measures derived from the census. The incentives contained in the agreements were expressed through, on the one hand, performance targets and indicators for several policy concerns, particularly the volume of services provided for public patients. On the other hand, if targets weren't met, there were clauses that could be invoked by the Commonwealth health minister for imposing penalties to reduce funding to the offending state. One consequence of this was that it provided an incentive for the states to conceal their performance, fudge their performance indicators and withhold information from the Commonwealth. This was so even if performance targets were going to be met, as there would always be some doubt about this in prospect.

In a major development, the 1993 Agreement created two bonus pools with formulas determining how they were to be disbursed. The formulas have an incentive structure which encouraged the states to do certain specified things to maximise their bonus payments. Defaulting on the supply of data necessary to calculate the bonus pool formulas was discouraged by clauses ensuring the partial distribution of the defaulting state's expected share of the bonus pool to the other states (Australian Government Solicitor 1993, Schedules D and J). The Commonwealth minister no longer had to exercise any discretion in all of this, and the result has been a complete change in the tactical possibilities available for funding variations under the agreements.

A sticking point in the negotiations was that the states found they could not calculate their expected bonuses in advance, and so claimed they could not decide whether to agree with the formulas for the bonus pools (Keith 1994). Eventually it had to be conceded that the point of bonus pools was that they could not be calculated in advance: this characteristic is of course necessary for them to function as incentives after the agreements have been entered into. The debate was thus forced to become one of the policy desirability of the incentive structure expressed by the bonus pool formula rather than the dollar amounts the states could expect.

The bonus pools were dropped from subsequent agreements, although strong financial incentives have been retained to encourage timely submission of performance data.

ADMINISTERING FREEDOM AND THE POLITICS OF MEDICARE

In a western democratic state such as Australia, policy debate and health system reform are threaded through and through with a concern for freedom of the public, health professionals and companies. Sometimes this concern is to restrict freedoms—for example, privacy laws that restrict the passing on of professionally acquired information about patients—and sometimes the concern is to preserve freedoms—for example, the way Medicare benefits effectively preserve a surgeon's ability to arrange treatment for their patient as the two of them see fit. Often, policies that provide freedoms to some types of actors in the health system necessarily place constraints on others. It could be said that the delineation of freedoms is one of the central necessities of health policy, and determines many of the ways in which health systems operate. The section includes a discussion of the way the governmental principles of democratic responsiveness and freedom of action are expressed in the governmentality of Medicare.

The introduction of Medicare has changed the democratic responsiveness of the health system in both a passive and an active sense. The technology of funding formulas actively utilises the enumeration of populations, so that the size, growth and health characteristics of the population—rather than their wealth, or political representation—are the most important determining factors in the distribution of resources for health. In this way, the population passively but powerfully affects the distribution of public sector health finances.

The advent of Medicare has also recast the possibilities and opportunities for health policy activism. The terrain within which people concerned with changing the health system stake out their ethical positions has changed. The development of funding formulas as a health financing technology has transformed the subjectivation of policy activists in the politics of health: it has raised new possibilities for reform; provoked new knowledges and new ways of making arguments; and allowed new, powerful connections to be made between health system financing and the ethical imperatives of democratic liberalism. It also created new objects for policy activists to turn their attention to: it reconstituted the population subjected to health services such that it actively and directly determines the distribution of resources; and reconstructed configurations of health care providers (such as general practice and the area health service) replete with policy levers to affect their style and practice of health care. I return to the discussion of policy activists in the final chapter.

Here I consider the incorporation of freedom of choice in health services in the Medicare system. This discussion illustrates how the introduction of Medicare dealt with the freedoms in the system concerning choice of doctor, choice of treatment and the freedom to insure.

In liberal societies, changes to the procedures of governing are introduced with respect to the value of freedom as it operates within society: 'the arts of government are systematically linked to the practice of freedom' (Rose 1992, p. 9). The introduction of Medicare as a new technology of government enhanced some freedoms within the health system and curtailed others. In the broad, soft footprint of Medicare's implementation, personal freedom to choose the health care that a person thinks they need has been enhanced; the freedom of doctors to treat patients as they think they need to be treated has been preserved; while the economic freedom of corporations involved in the financing of health care has actively been constrained and curtailed.

The introduction of Medicare provided greater freedom for members of the population to seek and receive health care, particularly for the 2 million people who did not have health insurance before Medicare was introduced. Apart from this change in access to services, the Commonwealth government introduced Medicare so as to have minimal visible impact on health care services, either with regard to the clinical freedom of health care professionals or with regard to the level of funding. The identified health grants and the Medicare grants to the states from 1983 onwards—the forerunners of the five-year funding agreements introduced from 1988—were varied to take into account historical hospital funding levels for this reason.

Concerning health financing, however, various freedoms were actively curtailed. All taxpaying persons were required to pay a Medicare levy on their taxable income to fund the increased cost to the government (not the total cost) of introducing the new arrangements, and insurance companies were stopped from offering insurance to cover medical costs. Doctors could continue to charge for their out-of-hospital services as they wished, although charges in hospitals were regulated by some state governments in response to the introduction of Medicare, notably in New South Wales through the amendments to the *Public Hospitals Act* that came into effect in early 1994. This Act made it a condition of appointment as a visiting practitioner that the practitioner should not charge more than the Commonwealth-controlled Medicare Benefits schedule for any service (Daniel 1990, p. 108) and was one of the precipitants of the dispute between the New South Wales government and public hospital doctors in 1984.

The introduction of Medicare changed the governmentality of the health system, but this also required a change in the government of freedoms associated with that system. The relation of the new health system to freedom of action displays three different gradients here regarding the type of actor and the type of freedom. Concerning actors, the freedom of individuals is enhanced; that of professionals is not changed; and that of corporations is curtailed. Concerning the type of freedom, freedom of access to health services is enhanced; freedom in the provision of clinical services is maintained; and freedom in arrangements for financing health care is curtailed.

These gradients in the government of freedoms in the health system related the economics of Medicare to the political maximisation of the electoral popularity of Medicare: it appealed directly to the public, many of whom were to benefit directly from it, with very few being out of pocket; it neutralised the professional concerns of doctors, thus stopping them from mobilising the public against the scheme, and restricting their own mobilisation to industrial concerns; and it offended the health insurers, who proved unable to significantly mobilise public sentiment against the reforms. In summary, the politics of the introduction of Medicare was a politics of freedom, not as a slogan or principle, but as the political management of a diverse set of freedoms among a diverse set of interest groups.

The main purpose of this chapter has been to examine themes in the political economy of the health system. The AHCA formula operates at the top of a cascade of funding arrangements in the Australian health system, and so is the logical point at which to examine the 'size of the pie'— that is, the makeup of total health expenditure in Australia. This chapter has traversed a series of issues in relation to this: long-term growth in health expenditure; the cross-section of expenditure across the public and private sectors; the transformations in expenditure patterns in each of these sectors, including the relations between public sector health expenditure and fiscal policy; and the relations between public and private sector health expenditures.

There is a general argument in economic circles that free market exchange between private individuals optimises the welfare of society: 'the prices that emerged from voluntary transactions between buyers and sellers—for short, in a free market—could coordinate the activity of millions of people, each seeking his own interest, in such a way as to make everyone better off' (Friedman and Friedman 1980, p. 32). Limiting this optimistic assessment of the power of markets is a further argument that it is true only in certain circumstances: 'A market is like a tool: designed to do certain jobs but unsuited for others. Not wholly familiar with what it can do, people often leave it lying in a drawer when they could use it. But then they also use it when they should not, like an amateur craftsman who carelessly uses his chisel as a screwdriver' (Lindblom 1977, p. 76). This conception underpins a research program, which commenced in the early 1960s, about the operation of health service markets and the clarification of what is referred to as 'market failure' in the health sector (Arrow 1963; McGuire et al. 1988). The argument goes that, in the face of market failure, the state legitimately can—and should—play a role in providing, or at least financing, health care.

The argument took a neo-liberal turn in the 1980s. On the one hand, against the earlier imaginary separation between private (market) and public (non-market) sectors in society, there was a recognition that the state created the conditions for markets to be established, and in a detailed way participated in the regulation and structuring of many (possibly all) particular markets. On the other hand, there were efforts to deploy market-type mechanisms—particularly price-based competition—in the distribution of public sector funds for the provision of public services. In the health sector, the Thatcher reforms to the National Health Service in the United Kingdom provide an example of the creation of such 'internal' markets (UK Department of Health 1989; Appleby 1992).

Rose provides a framework for understanding this neo-liberal turn by showing how the liberal (and neo-liberal) mode of government is concerned with understanding, delineating and mobilising various freedoms (for example, freedoms of belief, of choice, of action, of association) in the constitution of social activity (Rose 1992, 1993). Market mechanisms are just one of the technologies available for use within this governmentality; licensing is another (Osborne 1993). Rose emphasises that there are advantages and disadvantages, benefits and costs in the production and deployment of freedoms, and suggests a critical sociology of freedom to investigate both the techniques through which freedoms are produced and deployed, and the benefits and costs which accrue in relation to this mode of government. It is possible to see mainstream economic analysis of health care, which emphasises the failure of private markets and proposes state-controlled mechanisms in their place, as an example of such a sociology of freedom.

In my case studies of funding formulas in this and earlier chapters, I have tried to indicate the way in which the freedoms of those governed by the formula are central to the operation of the formula. More broadly, these analyses are an attempt to redress the weight of analysis of market mechanisms by offering an analysis of funding formulas as non-market, public sector resource-distribution mechanisms. I have not wanted to buy into the argument about whether funding formulas should replace market-based distribution of resources in the health sector. However, I have tried to show that they have. Large-scale public sector financing of health care services is likely to continue for the foreseeable future. The increasing sophistication of formula design that is evolving, along with the increasing availability of relevant data and the increasing capacity to mobilise these data within formulas, makes it likely that funding formulas will be used to distribute increasing portions of public sector health funding over the next decade. As indicated towards the end of the previous chapter, it is likely that a growth in expert knowledge and technical capacity within the public health disciplines will accompany this.

I would like to offer a few remarks on the nature of freedom within the neo-liberal mode of government. Neo-liberalism effectively repudiates the anti-government rhetoric of the twentieth century free marketeers such as Friedman and Hayek. For Friedman, society cannot continue indefinitely to sustain both private and public sector economic activity:

> in the words of Abraham Lincoln's famous 'House Divided' speech, 'A house divided against itself cannot stand . . . I do not expect the house to fall, but I do expect it will cease to be divided. It will become all one thing or all the other.' He was talking about slavery. His prophetic words apply equally to government intervention into the economy. Were it to go much further, our divided house would fall on the collectivist side. Fortunately, evidence is growing that the public is recognising the danger and is determined to stop and reverse the trend toward even bigger government (Friedman and Friedman 1980, p. 88).

There have been counter-arguments to this position since it was first articulated in Hayek's (1944) *The Road to Serfdom*: 'The freedoms that matter in ordinary life are definite and concrete; and they change with changing ways of different ages and civilizations . . . No one would suggest that all these freedoms are of equal importance; nor do these examples [given by Wootton] necessarily cover all the freedoms that we have, can have, or ought to have' (Wootton 1945, quoted in Hindess 1987, pp. 159–60). Such counter-arguments can be understood as forerunners of Rose's position, in that they problematise freedom as something to be analysed in its detail, rather than seeking to make a single, over-arching conception of freedom the central principle in a philosophy of government. At the heart of the debate—a debate that goes back at least to the seventeenth century—is the tension between freedom and determination. The precondition of free social action is the understanding that the effects produced by one thing are determined by the effects on it from other things. In other words, it is only by understanding the chains of causation between things that people can themselves cause things to happen that accord with their desires. Further, it is only by understanding the causes of their desires that people can truly be free. Freedom is thus located within the chains of causal determination, and is based in the most fundamental way on reason as the basis for understanding.

In Chapter 2, I attempted to show on the one hand how health operates as the precondition for freedom in the case of individual people, and on the other how health services have developed within a humanist project to increase the freedom of humankind through a variety of practical endeavours.

The two conceptions of freedom—Friedman's and Hayek's, versus Wootton's, Hindess's and Rose's—differ precisely in whether or not they recognise the practical nature of freedom. For the former, freedom has a primary, transcendental nature, and operates only as a unitary principle within social relations. It can be allowed to flourish or it can be constrained, which undermines the very condition of its existence, making it vanish in due course. For the latter, the dimensions of freedom are produced in many manifestations by many activities, including the work of rational reflection on the conditions of human existence, by the development of governmental technologies arising from this reflection into the concrete assemblages of society, and by the creative (and often unpredictable) responses to the social conditions that this governmental activity produces by the people it attempts to govern.

My analysis of various aspects of health financing has sought to demonstrate the merit of this practical view of freedom in relation to health policy. The study of the introduction of Medicare showed how the freedoms of patients were increased, those of doctors were not significantly altered, and those of private health insurance corporations were initially seriously curtailed in relation to insuring medical services, and were then later opened up to some extent through the allowance of 100 per cent cover and lifetime-rated products. The case study in the previous chapter on hospital funding showed how the New South Wales Resource Distribution Formula provides funding on a population health basis. While clinicians retain virtually a free hand in deciding what treatments to provide and who to treat, the formula exerts pressure on clinicians—and particularly clinician managers—to adopt population health thinking in making these decisions. The chapter on general practice documented the way a neo-liberal approach to funding general practice operates through the Practice Incentives Program formula, so that it is the free choices of patients and GPs that actually determine the value of payments made within the parameters of the formula.

In summary, these case studies have demonstrated the complex and widely distributed interplay between health service funding formulas and the subjective freedoms of actors in the health system, including the public. They have also demonstrated the independent fields of governmental action within which the three formulas studied operate. Certainly there are connections between them—for example, the AHCA formula funds the states, and New South Wales then applies this money to its RDF. But New South Wales adds in extra money to fund the RDF. It would be incorrect to see the cascade of formulas as forming a monolithic, integrated system of health financing. Each formula operates in a defined governmental space, with connections to others. The conceptual fields may share many features, and the strategic analyses of the agencies involved need to cover more than just the formula at hand.

These three chapters have attempted a pluralising analysis of funding formulas as a technology of government for distributing public sector resources. The value of a pluralising approach can be seen in relation to private sector markets as well: it is not helpful to see the world as consisting of a single, huge, integrated market. Even the analysis of global capital markets must proceed by examining the discrete and specific forms that these markets take and their separation from other markets for goods, services and money, notwithstanding the connections between these. There are myriad markets, more or less well defined, more or less connected to other markets and other spheres of social life. Similarly, it is not helpful to postulate that health system funding formulas for the distribution of public sector resources are, or will all be, drawn up into some mythical, totalising formula: they have been, and will be, established in many sites, for many purposes, bound up with the exercise of many freedoms in the widely distributed work of governing the health system.

7.

QUALITY AND SAFETY

QUALITY AND SAFETY IN THE HEALTH SYSTEM

This chapter turns to questions of the quality and safety of health care. Like many other industries, the health sector has engaged in a range of continuous quality improvement activities. Review of adverse events by clinicians with their colleagues is a particularly important activity for clinicians striving to do no harm to patients. Analysis of these activities brings out some interesting features of the relationship between clinical freedom and corporate accountability for health professionals in publicly funded health care settings.

There is a foundational divide in the health sector between the personal care of patients and the management of health care services. As discussed in Chapter 4, the personal care of patients is played out as a shepherd–flock game. The ethos of personal care is imagined through the idea of the well-trained health professional struggling against the arrows of disease and the slings of society with the best interests of the patient in mind. Opposed to this is the management of health care services, a city–state game where good managers provide facilities and support for patients and health professionals but don't interfere in the private practice of personal care. This model is seen in the image of hospital managers as overseeing the 'hotel services' of health care, and the insurance fund—public or private—that pays fees for any services, with no questions asked about those services' worth or appropriateness.

The science of medicine is closely focused on the personal care of patients. Investor-driven human science research is directed towards mass uptake of scientifically proven products through public financing and regulatory support for marketing permissions. Conversely, the analysis of health services management has a traditional focus on costs and efficiency. More recently, interest is emerging regarding how management and systems influence the quality and appropriateness of clinical care. Public health research is exploring methods to examine the impact of health system design on patient care and population health outcomes. These developments do not come from a U-turn in the ethos of either scientific medicine or public service in a liberal state. Rather, they come from a deepening of interests and methods: medical science has developed methods of investigating and testing the impact of social structures on human health, although many scientists are disappointed by the generalisability of such findings, as they are usually limited to the social contexts in which the investigations take place.

The quality movement in post Second World War industrial society analysed industrial manufacturing operations as social systems. Technologies of quality improvement proliferated, initially in manufacturing but also in service industries as these grew in economic importance. These technologies included standards and accreditation, quality circles, continuous quality improvement and total quality management. These have all been adopted in various ways in the health care sector. This has been driven by the financiers of health care, largely by government and public administration in Australia. The same anxieties that drove governments to increase their role in financing health care have also driven government action to assure quality of care in general and safety of care in particular.

Financier, and thus management, interest in quality improvement supplemented the traditional professional activities of training and collegiality associated with medical licensing. Doctors have been somewhat difficult to engage in management-driven quality initiatives; however, the profession has developed its own contribution to quality improvement technology. As foreshadowed in Chapter 5, population health techniques have become part of the stock in trade of clinical management. Peer review and clinical audit in essence take the ethos and techniques of the clinical sciences from their traditional application in the scrutiny of beneficial therapies and apply them to the scrutiny of adverse events. Special legal protections from litigation and prosecution have been provided by legislatures to give courage to clinicians so they will participate in these activities.

Starting with health financing, let's take a longer-term view. In the nineteenth century, health care was largely financed through point-of-service payments, including barter payment. Your physician provided you with a service and you paid him for it—particularly if you got better, although in general by the nineteenth century you paid for the service whether you got better or not.

Towards the end of the nineteenth century, a series of insurance systems developed where people arranged for their health care through mutual insurance. The development of friendly societies in Australia dates from that time. By sharing risk, people avoided financial ruin and helped their neighbours to avoid it too.

The state intervened in health financing, initially through the regulation of insurance and then, more recently in the post Second World War period, through the actual provision of health care financing from money raised through taxation. In Australia, 1996 was the first time there was a political consensus that the health system should be financed through taxation for universal care and access. That was the election in which John Howard's government was elected; it was health spokesperson Bronwyn Bishop who moved changes to the Coalition platform to support Medicare and so produce the bipartisan consensus. But that consensus had been coming in Australia since the Whitlam era, since the promise of Medibank in 1972. It could be argued that the party which has won government since then has always at least promised to provide a tax-financed health system for all, and that such a system has been the reality apart from the period from September 1981 to February 1984.

Why has this consensus on the role of state financing occurred? I have outlined the arguments from an economic and political perspective in earlier chapters. Here I would like to present them again from a managerial perspective, emphasising how best to serve the customers of a health service. One of the most telling reasons for state involvement is that, with health care, you cannot tell whether what you're spending your money on is worth it to you. When we book a holiday in Fiji, we think we know what value we will get for our money. When we actually take the holiday, we might think 'This place is not as good as it looked in the brochure' or 'I spoke to somebody else on the plane who bought their ticket for half the price that I paid', or we may have a fantastic time largely because of good weather. Essentially, we can judge the value of the holiday that we buy.

To personalise this, imagine the underlying conversation that takes place when a patient consults a surgeon. When you go to a surgeon and say, 'Doctor, I'm not feeling well', they may say, 'I'd like to cut you open'. Is that really going to make you feel better? We have to trust them, because we have no idea. There is so much expertise required, and the actual technologies of health care are so complex, that we cannot make our own purchasing decisions. Increasingly, this has led the populace right throughout the OECD to give a mandate to their governments to fund health services on their behalf. As a further development of the ethos that led to the mutual and friendly societies, this approach has enabled people to collectivise the formation of what they want from health care providers.

What does this have to do with quality and safety? Once the public had handed over a mandate to the state to provide health care services, they continued to accept the surgeon's advice to have an operation: 'I'm happy to have the operation if it really is going to make me better'. However, they also expected their government to ensure that the service was of a high quality. So what is quality? What are the dimensions of quality that people want? We want the services provided to be appropriate; we want our treatment to be effective; we want the service to be efficient because we don't want to pay more tax than we have to in order to have the government provide the health services for us. We want those services to be accessible— not just for ourselves, but for anybody else who is sick. We want them to be safe. And who's the we? The consumers are saying all this, so we can add that we want our services to be consumer driven.

Those are the dimensions of quality: appropriateness, effectiveness, efficiency, accessibility, safety and consumer focus. These dimensions come from the basic social contract of the public agreeing to hand over their taxes in exchange for a high-quality health care system. It's that expectation of a quality system that underpins the willingness to let the state arrange what to fund. If the public thought they could work it out for themselves and afford it themselves, they would. Because we don't really know what we need in terms of health care, we're happy to have the state take a role in order to ensure quality.

This same expectation of providing quality has developed for private insurance funding in the United States. There, the populace has not really demanded that health financing be provided through the states, except for the elderly and the indigent. Instead they have arranged for mutual insurance to provide their health care, but they still expect it to be of a high quality. That has underpinned the shift from benefits style schemes to managed care schemes that can answer the questions, 'Is it quality and is it what we need as a group of insured people?' In contrast, the Australian private health insurance fund managers have not as yet delivered on a commitment to quality. In time, however, I think they will increasingly be expected to ensure quality and safety in the services they finance. It is not good enough any more to say to your fund holders: 'leave that to the doctors'. The policy-holders are paying private health insurance companies as the policy providers to finance their health care for them, and they want them to ensure that the services provided are of a high quality.

In the nineteenth century, medical practice, midwifery and other early health professions were organised in cottage practices, operating as independent professionals. There were also the charity hospitals which had emerged in the eighteenth century, but whose numbers grew steadily throughout the world in the nineteenth century. By the twentieth century, we had networks of hospitals operated by religious organisations and governments. Towards the end of the twentieth century in Australia, regional health services became the dominant mode of organising health care services.

What has been behind this shift from cottage-based professionals and stand-alone charity hospitals to large, integrated regional health care organisations? The answer is that the increasing role of the state has led to the reorganisation of the health system in its own image, and the image of the state—or the organisation of the state—is according to democratic electorates. The politician's electorate became the region's population as the state took over responsibility for the provision of health care. The pressures on democratic governments, and the way that the state responds to pressure, are organised in population blocks (although the regional boundaries of the health system don't necessarily match the regional boundaries of the electorates). There are some other reasons for a drift towards regionalisation, but I think that is the main one.

What are the implications for safety and quality of this shift to regionalism? In the days of the independently operating hospital, the hospitals always strived for quality, ever since the advent of the scientific era. The higher the quality of the hospital—or at least their reputation—the more dangerous we expected them to be. That was where we expected the new operations to be tried, the new drugs to be tested, the new ways of managing things to be worked out. We accepted that increased danger of the high-reputation hospital because we thought it was important to drive progress.

Once ministers of state accepted responsibility for providing universal access to comprehensive health services in Australia, then responsibility for quality and safety loomed upon them. In the last decade, quality became a clear issue for the Australian Health Ministers Council. It created the Australian Council of Safety and Quality and Health Care, which reported directly to the ministers, coupled with allocating specific funds for safety and quality in the Australian Health Care Agreements (the major way that the Australian regional hospital networks are funded). In this way, health ministers grasped responsibility for quality and safety at the highest level. The Council for Safety and Quality in Health Care was constituted and tasked to create a greater desire for quality throughout the health system, and increase the motivation and means to pursue it at all levels. After five years, the council was superseded by the Australian Commission for Safety and Quality in Health Care, governed by the Australian Health Ministers Council.

In this diffused way, we are seeing quality and safety emerge as a bottom line for not just the ministers, but also for health departments and for regional health service agencies. One of the major themes in the analysis of governance of safety and quality has been that it has to be accepted at the top: responsibility must be taken at board level, or at general manager level, or at head of department level. For the public sector, management now makes the delivery of high-quality, safe health care a top priority. Traditionally, hospital managers took very little interest in clinical outcomes or the quality of care, but these days they are often at the top of a manager's performance agreement. This is reflected in their management of what we can call the clinical governance agenda and of the structures for clinical governance in regional health services. At the same time we have to keep in mind that, in the organisation of safety and quality, we must create and respect spheres of freedom in which practitioners can innovate. We have to give them the freedom to make their systems better at the same time as encouraging them not to tolerate readily preventable error.

Let us look briefly at another major part of our health system financing: our universal benefits schemes, the Pharmaceutical Benefits Scheme and the Medicare Benefits Scheme. Safety and quality are now central to the evolution of the Pharmaceutical Benefits Scheme. The PBS is an old scheme set up in the 1950s. As the state took responsibility for the universal provision of access to medicines, responsibility for safety and quality has been grasped firmly through the Quality Use of Medicines Program and the activities of the Therapeutic Goods Administration. The evolution of this responsibility is now taking place in the development of networked information technology to reduce medication error.

The Medicare Benefits Scheme, also dating back to the 1950s but achieving universal coverage only in the 1970s, has been much slower to address quality and safety. It does address quality in primary care through the Practice Incentives Program. However, in relation to specialist con-sultant practice and procedural practice, the Medicare Benefits Scheme has not grasped the safety and quality agenda at all. I think there is a clear opportunity there for the Commonwealth government to say they are going to start prescribing a bit of safety and quality through the Medicare Benefits that finance procedures. Given their responsiveness to the powerful financial incentives involved, the proceduralists certainly need a dose of it.

Through an analysis of the integration of purpose in the conduct of government, I have tried to show how the historical development of health financing has defined the dimensions of safety and quality in health care, and how the organisation of health services to serve well-demarcated populations has allowed safety and quality of care to emerge as a bottom line for ministers, managers and clinicians. In Chapter 5 I argued that the disciplines of public health—population science, epidemiology and the technologies of administration—have become central to health system management. These disciplines now support the pursuit of safety and quality in health care. Concerning expertise, the disciplines of public health are evolving techniques of investigation that support innovation in health service provision while paradoxically reducing tolerance of clinical practice variation by bringing error into stark relief. Concerning financing, there is further potential for private health insurance benefits and Medicare benefits for specialist consultations and procedures to be restructured to drive safety and quality.

CLINICAL GOVERNANCE

The increasing scrutiny of adverse outcomes and mistakes requires an evolution in the makeup of what we might call the professional conscience, specifically a greater willingness to provide constructive criticism to one's colleagues and to engage institutional managers in clinical care. The struggle of clinicians for the freedom to act in their patients' best interests is transformed as they become drawn into giving accounts of the quality and safety of clinical care to each other and to management. Conversely, corporate management is increasingly expected to ensure clinical governance is given as much attention as financial management.

This emerging nexus of accountability is transforming clinical freedom from negative freedom ('freedom from') to a positive freedom ('freedom to') (Berlin 1969). The traditional approach to clinical freedom has been to allow properly licensed doctors the freedom from constraint by any external authority on what they can do in their clinical practice. However, not only have these freedoms been constrained recently, but there have been extensive moves in many institutions to define what clinical privileges doctors have in that institution. A clinical privilege in this sense defines the positive freedom of what the doctor is allowed to do. The delineation of clinical privileges in this approach is based on the credentials that the doctor has, where the credential—usually a certification that the doctor has completed a particular course of study or supervised practice—provides a reasonable expectation that the doctor has the requisite expertise to safely do the procedures or manage the conditions that they have the clinical privileges to do.

Much of this style of approach to safety and quality in health care rests on the idea of adequate expertise within a scientific paradigm for health care. In the nineteenth century, medical science was investigating organs and tissues. Then, as the capacity to see smaller and smaller things developed, medical science moved down to the molecular structures.

In addition to this trend, in the post Second World War period we have seen the rise of the population sciences. Why did this happen? Why didn't medical science just continue its progress towards an atomistic view of health? I think there was a shift in the development of methods of observation from methods of seeing things better to methods of designing studies that showed us the relations between occurrences and let us examine causality. Part of the attraction of innovative study designs was a shift in the way that science was done. Scientists are free thinkers, and they need to be convinced to make up their own minds. The controlled trial enables them to look at health care interventions and say, 'well, that seems to actually work'. You don't need a more powerful microscope to run a controlled trial. You need a very careful method of study design.

In safety and quality (I say this as an epidemiologist, so take it with a grain of salt), with this shift towards population organisation of the health system and tax-based population financing of the health system, who were the scientists with whom the policy-makers and the politicians wanted to talk? They were population scientists. When the health department heads and health ministers ask about the scientific evidence, they don't want to know what the ion channel looks like. They want to know what the population studies have shown.

The same shift is happening in our teaching hospitals and medical schools. When I was a student, the professors were all people who were very good clinicians and also ran a wet lab. They knew about ion channels; they knew about the role of calcium in the regulation of blood pressure and could measure calcium concentration within subcellular structures. They knew about things at the molecular level. In contrast, the professors who have been appointed to the ANU Medical School in the twenty-first century need to be able to run clinical trials. This shift from wet lab to clinical trials expertise in academic clinicians has happened throughout the world.

In addition to clinical epidemiology, the technologies of government—administration and management—are also coming into focus as key research disciplines in the health sector. These are the social sciences that enable us to plan and test community-based, regulatory or administered interventions as we try to close the loop on the possibilities for improving patient care identified by clinical epidemiology.

Safety and quality in health care are related concepts. The main relationship is that both are pursued by continuous attention to the process of providing health care. Patient management plans and processes are often complex. Routine surgery such as hip replacement or coronary artery bypass grafting takes place through the provision of over 100 definable steps of care, from deciding the patient meets the indications for the procedure to post-operative review following rehabilitation. The chair of the Australian Council for Safety and Quality in Health Care (2000–05), Dr Bruce Barraclough, frequently commented that these processes were more complex than rocket science (a fair comment on a discipline that had last been at the cutting edge of technological endeavour in the 1960s).

Management of such complex patient management is itself an important process. If we remember the definition of government as the conduct of conduct, we can understand why the management of patient management processes is referred to as clinical governance. Clinical governance comprises many techniques drawn from a variety of fields and theories. It has assimilated many ideas from the systems theory developed in engineering and sociology in the mid-twentieth century, which has its roots in nineteenth century biology. Continuous quality improvement is based on the concept of the self-steering system, encountered in the concept of homeostasis in physiology, the self-correcting system in engineering, and the virtuous cycle in research policy (Wills 1999) (in contrast to the vicious cycle, another systems concept often used in political analysis). The continuous quality improvement cycle is based on clarification of the objective of the system, collection and review of data related to the components of the system, identification of problems, development and implementation of improvements, assessment of the impact on performance data, further identification of problems, and so on. The American statistician W.E. Demming is usually credited as the originator of postwar quality improvement culture, based on the part he played in the success of the Japanese manufacturing industry in the reconstruction effort in Japan under the Allied Forces Supreme Command. This approach was then introduced into the health sector, and received a significant boost from the visit to Australia by Brent James from Utah to provide training courses around the turn of the millennium. James's visit showed how quality improvement techniques could be combined with the clinical audit and peer review approach that was gaining popularity in the surgical disciplines. He taught root cause analysis, based on the identification and analysis of errors and adverse events, using techniques drawn from the field of aviation safety (James 2005).

How does this all fit together? Continuous quality improvement projects, peer review and clinical audit, as professional activities conducted at the local level, can be understood as the broad base of the regulatory pyramid that has been described by John Braithwaite, a sociologist at the Australian National University (Braithwaite, Makkai and Braithwaite 2007; Braithwaite and Drahos 2000). Up from these activities, in the middle of the pyramid, are a series of regulatory interactions with the state, including registration of health professionals, health facility licensing, complaint investigation and reparation systems. At the top of the pyramid is the regulatory power to ruin a practitioner or health care operator—for example, by removal of their licence to practise, heavy fines or a gaol sentence.

Braithwaite and colleagues have extensively investigated regulatory systems. They have concluded on the empirical evidence that regulatory systems work best when they have the pyramidal structure described above. They are considerably less effective if they lack either the broad base of self-regulatory quality improvement activities or a sharp apex of ruinous powers.

Of themselves, strong regulatory powers may achieve high compliance with simple measures—for example, the threat of deregistration is sufficient to cause the great majority of physicians to pay their annual registration fees. However, a regulatory scheme with strong powers to ruin, but without effective broad-based activity, has little chance of translating the teeth into effective improvements in care. It may happen, but it will be haphazard and cannot be expected to succeed in any systematic way. On the other hand, a regulatory scheme that relies on well-developed, broad-based activity without strong powers of ruination, that can be deployed when necessary, suffers from widespread lack of compliance with broad-based improvement activity and a tendency for issues to escalate up to the next level of regulatory stringency. In turn, this can overload the higher regulatory mechanisms, which have serious difficulty resolving the large number of issues referred. Enforcement officers at higher levels of the regulatory scheme who do not have a real pointy end available to them get caught between turning a blind eye or demonstrating their impotence.

A regulatory schema with a sharp apex on top of a well-developed pyramid of broadening activity with decreasing sanctions operates in the opposite way: the threat of ruin drives energetic efforts to resolve things before they escalate, and there are well-developed structures within which to do this.

Hospital accreditation illustrates this well. The Australian Council on Healthcare Standards (ACHS) hospital standards and accreditation scheme is itself a regulatory activity in the middle of the pyramid. When it operated in isolation in the 1980s, it had a limited capacity to improve quality in the hospital system. However, when combined with performance agreements around achieving accreditation for senior managers (including the threat of career termination), peer review activities required by professional associations such as the Royal Australasian College of Surgeons, and extensive self-assessment activities in the inter-accreditation period, the ACHS scheme has been built into a much more comprehensive regulatory pyramid with much wider impact and effectiveness. In the Australian Capital Territory, accreditation has been linked to hospital licensing. If a hospital loses its accreditation, it is required to undergo regular audits by the licensor (the Chief Health Officer). Failing an audit against the ACT Health Facilities Code of Practice results in loss of licence. Without a licence, the facility is not allowed to treat patients.

QUALITY OF CARE AND POPULATION HEALTH

One of the reasons why change in safety and quality in health care has happened so slowly is because it has been very hard to capture and marshal the clinical information required to actually demonstrate the quality and safety of the health care system. However, information technology developments that are happening now are finally allowing managers to see the quality and safety of the operations they are managing. Once moderate visibility of this is achieved, many more gains will follow.

The gains in population health outcomes from safety and quality will come from some specific sources. One is better case-finding of people who are at risk, and better monitoring of people's needs. This can be illustrated by considering people with Type II diabetes. The Australian estimates are that 50 per cent of people with Type II diabetes in Australia have not been diagnosed (Barr et al. 2006). If you can find these people, you can offer them care earlier and stop their complications developing. Once they've been found, it is also possible to monitor their needs. If people have diabetes and we're following them, we can check, for example, how their blood sugar control is going over the course of the year. How are their retinas—are they at risk of going blind? Should they have preventative laser surgery? Better monitoring of people with treatable chronic illness leads to significant improvements in quality of life.

A second set of gains will come from delivering the right care to the right patients at the right time, every time. We have the technology and we have the clinicians to deliver really good care for a very wide range of conditions. For example, at Calvary Hospital, a public hospital with a district level emergency department in the Australian Capital Territory, they found that only one-third of patients presenting with a myocardial infarction were getting the right treatment—which is blood thinners—within two hours of arrival. So they undertook a quality project which lifted that rate to 93 per cent, and they're now one of the country's leaders in the best practice care for people presenting with myocardial infarction. It has made a huge difference in terms of lives saved and in morbidity avoided for those people, and there's been no change in technology. The only change is that the right care is being provided to the right patients every time now. Calvary has become a benchmark for myocardial infarction treatment across the country (Penman and Dugdale 2003, p. 50). There are many similar examples relating to medication management of other conditions. Accurately targeted procedures and better medication management, coupled with the right procedure for the right patient, reduce adverse events and enhance health outcomes.

How does this look from an epidemiological perspective? To take my own jurisdiction, of the total deaths in the Australian Capital Territory for the year 2000, about 25 per cent were avoidable. Within that 25 per cent, we can avoid one-third of the cardiovascular deaths. We can also avoid maybe one-fifth of the cancer deaths that we are seeing, and a smaller number of respiratory deaths. Many of the remaining preventable deaths come from accidents and injuries. These areas are where we can find the gains (Dugdale and Kelsall 2004).

Let's also look at life expectancy at birth for women and men from 1971 to 2001. Life expectancy for men in 1971 was about 68 years. That wasn't very long ago. Now it's about 78 years. I remember in the early 1990s being up to my neck in health policy. I had no idea that we were supposed to be delivering improvements in life expectancy. I thought we'd got all those. Now I look at the gains and say to myself: 'Well, what are we going to do over this decade to continue to deliver those gains in life expectancy?'

Improving infant mortality is another way. Gains in infant mortality have been dramatic, and place us as one of the best jurisdictions in the entire world. Again, look at the trend. We've got to keep delivering on this—because we can.

We must also look at the death rates, the flip side of the picture. This is really what we're working on—just really pushing down the death rates for babies, men and women. The trend is downwards, but can we continue it? Practically, I think the public's health can continue to improve. The public system is expected to deliver, and is acquiring the techniques and the governance—the clinical governance—to actually focus on the delivery of more health gains for the population.

It is population science techniques that we use to monitor this, and to help direct the effort into exactly where it is needed. We haven't invented a new mode of treatment—for example, the great majority of the people presenting at Calvary Hospital in Canberra with myocardial infarction were given life-saving blood thinners within two hours of arrival. That outcome comes thanks to quality systems, through better clinical governance. A small additional gain can be achieved by arranging access to emergency angioplasty for some of these patients. In Canberra, this was initially achieved by building on the rapid assessment approach for patients presenting at Calvary with chest pain, and adding rapid transport to the angioplasty suite at the tertiary hospital 20 minutes away by ambulance.

Why am I optimistic that these trends will continue? I think the information and communication technology for health that has been implemented from the early 1990s right through to now—indeed, implemented in a very profound way—will accelerate those gains over the next decade. So, even though there may be fewer health gains to extract, I think we'll get much of them over the next decade.

INFORMATION AND COMMUNICATION IN HEALTH CARE

When making clinical decisions, clinicians bring together specific and general information relevant to the patient and their condition. This bringing together of relevant information is frequently a difficult and complex task. As general medical knowledge has grown, the difficulty and complexity of having the right knowledge and information at hand has increased. Because of the limitations of human intellectual and memory capacity, this growth in knowledge has driven increasing specialisation, breaking the field of clinical practice down into small enough fields so that clinicians in that super-specialty could reasonably be expected to have a strong clinically relevant knowledge about it and have access at their fingertips to current and emerging knowledge.

A related strategy that has been used to deal with the increasing complexity of information wrangling for clinical decision-making has been to increase the time clinicians spend educating themselves. Throughout most of the twentieth century, medical training comprised six years of undergraduate study. On top of this, compulsory supervised internships were introduced first in Queensland in 1940 (Gillespie 1991, p. 79) and later throughout Australia. By the 1980s, around half of all medical practitioners had gone on to do specialty training, usually through five years of supervised practice and study supervised by the relevant specialty college. In the 1990s, the Commonwealth legislated so that from the late 1990s new graduates needed to obtain postgraduate specialty qualifications (including in general practice, itself a specialty) in order to be recognised for the payment of Medicare benefits. In the last decade, specialist medical colleges and some state medical registration boards have required doctors to undertake continuing medical education once they have obtained their specialty qualification. Medicine has always been a profession with an ethic of lifelong learning, but this was often observed in the breach. The increasing complexity of health care has meant that this has now become *de rigueur*.

A further strategy is also emerging. Developments in information and communications technology, particularly with the advent of networks of computers, are facilitating the presentation of precisely the right general medical information with precisely the right patient information at the time and place of decision-making. For example, most general practitioners now use clinical software that combines patient notes with electronic prescription writing. When composing the prescription on the computer, the software will pop up information about such things as interactions with other drugs the patient is on, or advise reducing the dose because of the patient's age.

There are two types of information that need to be brought together for clinical decision-making: particular information concerning the patient about whom the decision is being made; and general information relating to the disease or therapy under consideration. The particular information includes the patient's age, gender, medical history including diagnoses and medications they are taking, physiological parameters such as blood pressure, height, weight, and so on. The general information includes results of trials of interventions relevant to the patient's condition, protocols for management agreed by relevant expert associations, medication regimes agreed between pharmaceutical manufacturers and regulatory authorities, and adverse events to be watched for. Health professionals bring together these two types of information in their clinical reasoning. Each type of information has its associated textual form: particular information is written down in the clinical notes; general information is published in journals and textbooks. Recently, as computers became ubiquitous, software programs have been developed to facilitate making clinical notes, and textbooks, journals and expert advice have been published on the internet.

Clinical notes software rapidly developed into the clinical desktop, the computer version of the doctor's desk on which the patient's notes are opened, the doctor's key textbooks or pocket guides are standing and in front of which are pinned guidelines from their colleagues (e.g. the list of diseases that must be notified and the address for notification; consensus guidelines for managing a condition commonly seen in the practice; a research protocol for a trial in which the doctor is participating).

The next major development, now underway, is for the clinical desktop to be connected to a network, or a network of networks, so that it can marshal particular patient information from a wide range of sources, including other clinicians' notes, hospital admission and discharge information, medications prescribed and dispensed, diagnostic test results, X-ray images, and so on. Similarly, for general information the computer desktop should be able to marshal, from trusted internet sources, up-to-date clinical evidence and consensus guidelines relevant to that patient at the time of consultation. Currently, clinical desktops participate in ad hoc networks. The challenge for clinical computing is to systematically network the clinical desktops of all clinicians dealing with more or less well-defined patient populations. If we take the example of Australians eligible for Medicare, this would mean that, on the one hand, all clinicians would be networked and use electronic health records that can be read by any other clinician seeing the same patient (if the patient consents to this) and, on the other hand, the network would include servers providing recognised clinical guidelines so that the clinical desktop software can draw down the appropriate part of the guideline at the appropriate time.

Such integration of patient information and clinical guidelines, and their presentation to the clinician at the place and time of clinical decision-making, require that participating clinical desktops, electronic health records and clinical guidelines can recognise the relevant parts of each other through information architecture approaches such as adherence to style standards, shared terminologies and ontologies of clinical practice, and common use of higher order programming languages such as HL7 (Health Language 7), and that participating computers communicate with each other through standardised communication protocols. Security, privacy and access to records need to be controlled to a similar level as computerised banking. The right parts of the participating guidelines would need to be readily findable, with clinical desktops keeping open a Google-like search for keywords, diagnoses and classes of patients to whom the guidelines apply, with the desktop bringing these close to the open page as the clinician moves towards making a decision.

The health sector spends about 2 per cent of its total expenditure on information and communications technology (ICT). That is well below the average for other technologically driven sectors of the economy. If it were in education, mining or hospitality and tourism, it would be more like 5 per cent—that's a fairly average ICT spend for a service industry.

Why is the health sector lagging behind in the adoption of information and communications technology? I think one answer is that there is a lot of tradition in health. We have large institutions which are partially closed and which change only very slowly. The second problem, paradoxically, is that the health sector has a very high level of functionality in information processing and in communication using traditional methods.

We have an excellent method of communicable disease notification based on faxes. It's simple. It's been set up for many years and it works very well. So if anyone wants to talk to us about getting with the modern world, we respond that we believe in what we're doing and sometimes question the fallibility of modern electronic systems. Is there sufficient robustness in these new systems for us? We already know the fax system is very robust. It's a similar argument with clinical communication. People in the X-ray business took a fair bit of convincing that the electronic delivery of a film of an X-ray on a video unit was going to be better than actually getting the plastic film and holding it up to the light. In fact, this has now happened for much of radiology, particularly with the advent of digital image capture and computerised image processing. Lost films and repeat X-rays have been significantly reduced.

The health system has a high level of functionality that makes people get quite concerned about adopting new technology. However, one of the things that marks the health sector is that when it does adopt new technology, it does it quickly and very well. When I first moved into the Commonwealth Department of Health, people would say to me: 'No offence to you, but your colleagues are just so conservative and it's so hard to change anything.' I replied that it was just not true. They're hard to convince, but look at the way they respond to clinical evidence. When the drug companies made the drug class of statins available for the treatment of high cholesterol, doctors were quite sceptical. But once the evidence was in, and they saw them work—saw them produce lower cholesterol levels—the adoption of statins by the medical profession was unbelievably rapid. It took all of the bureaucrats by surprise, which meant their budgets blew out by factors of several times what the expectations were.

The same has happened with angioplasty. Angioplasty in the early 1990s was used on a very small percentage of patients with blockages in their arteries. But as the techniques improved, and as the angioplasty pro-ceduralists were able to demonstrate that they could actually make the gain for that patient's health and avoid an open heart procedure, the number of angioplasties has risen as quickly as the angioplasty suites where the procedure takes place could be built.

There are a number of other examples we could cite. The pattern in health seems to be that people are initially sceptical but become rapid adopters once the switch that allows them to appreciate the evidence has been tripped. This is a pattern of stability punctuated by rapid change. And once we decide to change, we do it very well.

I think that we're at that point now with information and communications technology for health. Patients and clinicians expect much better communication now than they did even ten years ago. It is now not good enough for a patient to turn up in a specialist's surgery without their results or without the specialist being able to get ready access to the results. It's no longer good enough for them to come into hospital and find the admitting intern has to repeat all their tests because they haven't got them with them. The patients say: 'I've told the doctor. I've had that test—can't you get the results?' Patients and clinicians now expect better service, having seen other aspects of society where there's very fast communication.

Chronic disease management requires much better information and continuity of information. Management of diabetes, for example, requires surveillance from diagnosis through to death. Good surveillance and monitoring should be used to adjust treatment and reduce the rate of progression of complications. That's the pattern for most chronic diseases—information will allow better management and better quality of life—but it's also the case for episodic hospital care for the patient being admitted for an operation.

One of the key changes here is the rise of day-of-surgery admission. In times gone by, the idea was you came in a day or two before surgery and we'd sort you out and make sure everything was in order. These days, we're aiming for at least three-quarters of patients who are having surgery to come in on the day of admission. For this to occur, everything needs to be sorted out in advance and communicated to the hospital and to the right parts of the hospital on the day of surgery, because within two or three hours of hitting the hospital you're under anaesthetic and having a procedure.

Pressures from patients and from the business of what we are doing, combined with the availability of information and communications technology, are driving the health system towards a fully interlaced clinical information and communications environment. In Australia, the governments of the states, territories and the Commonwealth have joined together to form a company called the National E-Health Transition Authority (NEHTA). The major areas in which NEHTA is introducing standards and pathways for information technology transformation are supply chain management, integration of communication standards between hospitals and other agencies, secure messaging and information transfer, consent models that address the issues of privacy and access to information, development of indexes and directories so patients and clinicians can find each other's data, and of course standards for the clinical data themselves.

Once these building blocks are in place, it will allow full communication between all the different clinicians and units working within the health care system. From the patient's point of view, it all ends up in an event summary of their health record, although that health record itself need not ever be held comprehensively together in one single location.

However, in order to gain the health value from the investment in information and communications technology, data-handling capacity needs to be combined with expert decision-support systems. These are developing in quite a piecemeal fashion, with a myriad of groups developing care protocols and guidelines, and all publishing them on the internet. I expect that, over the next few years, we will see development of a policy agenda to integrate these systems into the operation of the health system at the level of the clinical desktop.

To understand the governmentality surrounding safety and quality of health care, we should keep in mind that it is the counter-intuitive character of health care which has driven the transformation towards state financing and state organisation of health care. This transformation has privileged the population sciences in public management, and established safety and quality of health care as a bottom line to obtain the greatest population benefit out of the health system. The same motivation is now driving investment in information and communications technology, although the health sector has been slow to adopt this—possibly in part due to the lack of market-based drivers for technology adoption in a largely government-funded system, and in part due to the conservatism of the medical profession. However, this transformation is now underway, and will contribute to drawing closer together the data-hungry population sciences with hospital and area-based health service provision.

8.

DOING INDIGENOUS HEALTH POLICY

Paul Dugdale and Kerry Arabena*

AUSTRALIA'S INDIGENOUS HEALTH POLICY CONTEXT

The health of Aborigines and Torres Strait Islanders is poorer than that of the general community on most indicators, as is the case for the indigenous populations in other liberal democratic countries. Poor indigenous health status has long been recognised as a health policy problem at the international, national and state levels. While much has been done here, resulting in improvements in the health status of Indigenous Australians over the last decades, a significant gap has remained in the health status between Indigenous Australians and other people in Australian society. This life expectancy gap is not now as wide in other countries such as Canada, the United States and New Zealand, where significant reductions in health inequalities between the indigenous and general populations have occurred over the last 20 to 30 years (Kunitz 1996).

Indigenous peoples, health practitioners, policy planners, funding agencies and advocacy bodies have all expressed the view that Australia can

---

* Kerry Arabena has been the chief executive officer of the Apunipima Cape York Health Council, the Pintubi Homelands Health Service (the most remote Aboriginal Medical Service in Australia) and the Sexual Health and Family Planning ACT Health Service (a mainstream service where she worked closely with Paul Dugdale). At the time of writing, she is a Visiting Research Fellow in Social Health at the Australian Institute of Aboriginal and Torres Strait Islander Studies and the Cooperative Research Centre for Aboriginal Health.

do significantly better on Indigenous health. International experience has shown that health improvements in marginalised indigenous communities are achievable given a clearly expressed political will for this to happen, and sufficient money. In Australia, policy frameworks and health strategies have not been easy to coordinate for the benefit of all Aboriginal and Torres Strait Islander peoples. Some programs have worked extremely well, such as the elimination of Hansen's disease (leprosy) in the Top End, the delivery of surgery for blindness along with treatment and prevention of trachoma in arid communities, and the creation of a network of community-controlled Aboriginal Medical Services (AMSs) across the country. Other health initiatives have not lived up to expectations, however.

It is important to consider the overall policy context in which Aboriginal and Torres Strait Islander health improvements are to be achieved. On 15 April 2004, the Howard government announced that it was introducing significant changes to the delivery of services to Aboriginal and Torres Strait Islander people, distributing across all relevant government departments the responsibility to implement coordinated programs for Indigenous Australians through a whole of government approach. The emphasis on improving the performance of the public sector through the adoption of processes variously called 'whole of government approach', 'joined up' government or 'connecting government' saw the trialling of the integration of policy development, service delivery, engagement with communities and a focus on achieving outcomes. These approaches were expected to inspire national approaches to the delivery of services to Indigenous Australians, and people implementing these new approaches were required to commit to the implementation of the policy frameworks. It was believed these and other types of government initiatives had the potential to overcome the disadvantage experienced by Indigenous Australians and to effect inter-generational change.

At the same time as this redesign of public infrastructure, the Commonwealth government abandoned national and regional representative structures for Aboriginal and Torres Strait Islander people. In the regional sense, these representative structures were hubs with which government agencies could consult and engage Aboriginal and Torres Strait Islander peoples in activities that affected health and other outcomes in cross-jurisdictional areas. The 2004 policy changes thus severed all legitimate links between governments and their constituents, requiring a rethink of how to broker health improvements with Indigenous people across the country.

Our federal health system has, at best, under-performed in the area of Aboriginal health and facilitated mainstream programs that are often inaccessible to Indigenous peoples. In any administrative context, there are opportunities to enhance health outcomes for Aboriginal people through policy formation and program delivery. Since 2004, efforts have been made to reduce administrative barriers, undertake innovative approaches, address community need and improve government coordination to bring about changes in Aboriginal and Torres Strait Islander peoples' health status.

Developing workable solutions still requires the standard policy toolbox, including consultation, data analysis, program design and evaluation capabilities. However, the new policy environment introduced by Howard has given rise to specific challenges to the rights of Indigenous peoples. Accepting responsibility for appropriate engagement and designing policies and programs that are accessible to Indigenous communities is paramount. As is often the case, the failures of government and other health service delivery agencies are most keenly experienced by the most vulnerable and marginalised in a society, not those who implement them.

There are structural pressures for government agencies, and non-government agencies that are funded by governments, to reduce or abandon collegial forms of deciding what to do. This has been exacerbated in recent years by the implementation by government departments of a particular legal form of accountability based on a specific form of managerialism. This is an amalgam of 'management by objectives', popularised by the success of California's Silicon Valley pioneer Hewlett-Packard, combined with what has been called 'the New Contractualism' (Davis, Sullivan and Yeatman 1996) where government funding for non-government organisations was shifted from grants to contracts with a concomitant reduction in flexibility, and an increase in reporting and audit requirements. A good example is the changes in the administration of the Community Development Employment Projects following the abolition of the Aboriginal and Torres Strait Islander Commission, and the transfer of administrative responsibility for CDEP to the Department of Employment and Workplace Relations (Sanders 2007).

While there are advantages to this type of administrative technology, it is prescriptive in the way that contractually funded agencies and organisations can operate and help people. It can also pressure people within the funded organisations to lose touch with the community they are supposed to serve, because they develop their own need to succeed and be perceived as successful by the bureaucracies to which their government contracts hold them accountable.

As a part of the new contractualism within a politicised public service, the underlying obligation to serve the public can be displaced by a duty to be politically obsequious. Contracts by their very nature are drawn up because the parties to them do not trust one another. When Aboriginal organisations deal with the state and the bureaucracy, they rarely feel that anyone is listening to them dispassionately, in a dialogue of equals. The dialogue is instead a negotiation to enter a contractual obligation to participate in a civilising project, not a recognition of the value of self-determination. Organisations with contracts are expected not to criticise the government, and if they do they can expect to be discriminated against in future tenders and contract negotiations. It is difficult being subversive when dealing with Indigenous affairs. The world as it is now doesn't appreciate subversiveness as a technique or as a motivation, and it can put other people at great risk. People dissenting from the bureaucracy place themselves at risk of marginalisation and intolerance. This is true for people within the bureaucracies as well.

The delivery of health care to Indigenous populations of people has been bound up in the red tape of the new contractualism, with some AMSs having over 40 separate contracts with government at the one time. Rather than tying them up with a politically motivated surfeit of accountability, there is a good case that, given the success of AMSs in providing primary care to Indigenous communities, and the consensus on the need to expand primary care, the Commonwealth government-funded growth in these services should have been significantly higher than it has been over the last fifteen years.

In most OECD countries with a colonial history, apart from Australia, the colonising governments have some sort of foundational treaty with their indigenous people. This provides a constitutional and legal framework within which negotiations and contractual arrangements can and should occur, notwithstanding that this has often been observed in the breach. The Australian state was constituted in a way that excluded Indigenous people from sharing in the benefits flowing from nationhood (Anderson 2007). This has partly been rectified by constitutional amendments (culminating in the 1967 amendments), the *Aboriginal Land Rights (Northern Territory) Act 1976*, similar Acts in other states, and by the *Mabo* judgment recognising native title in Australian common law (Mason et al. 1992) and the

Native Title Act 1995. However, conferring citizenship and the recognition of land ownership by Indigenous people are only starting points. These legal events within the colonising state create the conditions of possibility for equitable negotiations over property and the benefits of citizenship.

Concerning government services, if Australia is going to have legal agreements with Indigenous people based on that identity and account-ability contracts as the fundamental basis of the relationship between bureaucracies and Indigenous citizens, then these notions should be framed in a way that gives everyone the opportunity to have some input regarding what the principles, values, agreement-making processes and end result of those processes should be. Without a mutually understood framework for the state's dealings with, say, community-controlled organisations, services to Aborigines will continue to stultify.

This chapter examines some of the major themes of this book in relation to Indigenous health policy. It begins by considering the Commonwealth government framework and administrative mechanisms that shape Indigenous health policy. It then explores the nature of health and its relation to freedom in a case study about the relations of art to health care in the Western Desert. It concludes by considering how we can move on from an understanding of the social determinants of health to create a real determination to achieve better health.

Public policy formulators and implementers are responsible for the health outcomes of large numbers of people, with national approaches providing a health and well-being framework in which up to 20 million people are engaged. This can be difficult to conceive. Making policy creates major changes to the conditions within which people live their lives. For policy-makers doing work on settings with which they are familiar, their background store of taken-for-granted understandings of everyday life makes a valuable contribution to their policy work. What is not well under-stood is how non-Indigenous people can best work with Indigenous people in rural, remote and urban settings. Policy planners and others need to include in their suite of public policy tools a process of appropriate, spatially distributed consultation with Indigenous communities that is based on cross-cultural understandings, respectful communication and background research to give issues depth and insight.

Policy is often formed initially around analysis that imagines a static structure with a mechanistic focus in its implementation. Following this, in the struggle around the creation of the policy (i.e. when trying to get it agreed to by the various agencies that participate in it actually becoming law), politics and money intrude. In this context, questions arise about who will be the winner in terms of increasing their freedom and power to act, and who is going to lose because their power to do things is constrained. That happens at two levels: both within the bureaucracy where power struggles are endemic, and in the field where the policy is to be applied. These struggles can actually reduce the overall health benefits for constituents as, instead of working collaboratively, there is competition to determine the winners and losers. As they say in the Torres Strait, some days you eat the crocodile and some days the crocodile eats you.

UNIVERSAL AND HOLISTIC IDEAS OF HEALTH

The various ideas of health discussed throughout this book are essentially part of a European discursive tradition that dominates thinking about health policy in Australia. For Indigenous people, it is becoming increasingly difficult to articulate the need for health to be achieved in a distinctive reality with distinctive values in the context of land, and not in the context of a European modernity. 'Eurocentricity' in this sense is more problematic than may at first be thought. If Europe is the paradigm for modernity, we are all—European and non-European—to a degree inescapably Eurocentric (Chaudhuri 2004). An examination of the nature of health is required. More consideration is needed as to the meaning of health and health care for Indigenous people. An understanding of the nature of health is an important consideration for policy and for program implementers in the field.

If health care is conceived as services provided to people across their lifetime, with specific interventions targeting individuals in utero, at birth, through childhood, adulthood and old age, Aboriginal and Torres Strait Islander health care has improved and become more effective over the last 30 years. Whether a health service implements health promotion programs or clinical interventions, much of health service delivery has been about wanting people to be well, to have good health and a quality of life that will facilitate 'Indigenous people being able to share in the benefits and the bounty that Australia brings to all its citizens' (Howard 2005).

The health care system in Australia is underpinned by ideas about the universality of health, about health for the whole. It has widely been assumed that services with a theoretical underpinning of universal health could benefit all Australians and overcome their particularity, no matter the social or group differences, or the inequalities in wealth, status and power. This is not the case. Universal aspirations are not enough, particularly for Indigenous peoples. On the contrary, the concept of universality can suppress the variety of identities and in effect silence, stigmatise and marginalise groups and identities that lie beyond the boundaries of the mainstream (Beiner 1995, p. 9). In this way, universal health concepts are a cover for a particular approach which Indigenous peoples cannot readily accept or embrace.

What often happens is that Aboriginal and Torres Strait Islander people are accused of not wanting health, or being incapable of looking after themselves, or they are made responsible for health by policy-makers, funding agencies and services which are not concerned with where or how Indigenous peoples might be able to articulate their own concepts of health. Often Indigenous peoples are marginalised and stigmatised, labelled and blamed for their lack of participation in service systems that in many cases perpetuate a colonial experience. As pointed out by Senator Aden Ridgeway, one of Australia's few Indigenous parliamentarians, in his valedictory speech:

> Defining us as 'disadvantaged citizens' masks the structural and systemic barriers that have contributed to the situation we now find ourselves in and it enables the debate and proposed solutions to be grossly over-simplified. We need to be careful not to be co-opted into over-simplified debates about our needs which are based on language which is benign in appearance, but loaded in meaning (Ridgeway 2005).

The commonsense view inherent in the language of colonialist health agendas disregards different truths espoused by Indigenous peoples and others, or casts them as lesser truths. Language constructs the sense of privilege that pervades European modernity (Aldrich 2006).

With an overwhelming majority of 143 votes in favour, only four negative votes cast (Canada, Australia, New Zealand, the United States) and eleven abstentions, the United Nations General Assembly adopted the Declaration on the Rights of Indigenous Peoples on 13 September 2007. The declaration has been negotiated over 20 years between nation-states and indigenous peoples. This declaration recognises the health concepts of indigenous individuals as having the right to life, physical and mental integrity, liberty and security of person. All of the articles in the declaration, including those focusing on self-determination, governance structures, access to education and technology, the right to non-discrimination and to describe oneself as belonging to a particular group of people, are aimed at enhancing the health and well-being of indigenous peoples across the world (United Nations 2006). The resolution marks the recognition throughout the world of an indigenous perspective on these matters.

Aboriginal and Torres Strait Islander people in Australia often describe health in a holistic way—in that it is simultaneously intuitive and rational, scientific and artistic. Such concepts explain the view of Indigenous health focusing on prevention and clinical interventions with complementary issues such as substance misuse, housing, employment, justice, policing and strengthening cultural connections. These health ideals are documented in the recommendations of a series of reports that, while never fully implemented, remain powerful aspirational statements about holistic health. Examples of these ideals are included in reports such as those that resulted in the Aboriginal Deaths in Custody Report (Johnston 1991) and the Stolen Generations Report (HREOC 1997).

Holistic health interventions have become generally accepted in the public domain, but are yet to be effectively coordinated in government departments, other health agencies and within communities. But Aboriginal people have at the same time become limited by the way these broader conceptions remain fixed on personal and community well-being. This makes it difficult for Indigenous people who want to assert health and well-being as referent to something other than a colonial experience. It seems inescapable. Colonisation is an instrument of domination and a central principle of modernity, the ongoing experience of which is profoundly European in Australia, Canada, America and New Zealand, as well as other countries.

These health concepts, and the colonial-referent politics and policy manoeuvrings, shape the debate and discussion about Indigenous affairs in a way that takes for granted the oppression and marginalisation of Indigenous people within the Australian state. In this way, Aboriginal and Torres Strait Islander peoples are beholden to government, which determines whether we can control our own affairs. This determination is dependent on society's views of our competence in terms that describe our contributions to the market economy, not in terms of what it might be that Indigenous peoples can offer all citizens in Australia.

This is manifested as identity politics. The ascription of identifying characteristics is the principal starting point from which a non-Indigenous health professional can describe and engage politically with Indigenous health issues. This gives Indigenous people limited scope to mobilise their other experiences or other world views into discussions and debates with non-Indigenous health professionals. It discourages Indigenous people from insisting on the practices and understandings that form Indigenous peoples' ways of life as something to value, and that cannot be subsumed into western conceptions of well-being. As stated by Martin Nakata, 'our philosophies or world views cannot simply be re-explained or re-interpreted by informed, educated or expert people outside of our communities. To do so is a negation or denial of our experience and our understanding of our own position as we confront alien—and alien-ating—practices and knowledge' (Nakata 2007, p. 8).

The identity politics of Indigenous struggles is the accepted mantle an Aboriginal person takes on to assume an advocacy role for health advancement or health achievement in Australia. Fundamentally, identity politics divides Indigenous people and other Australians into separate communities of 'us' and 'others'.

In a referendum on 27 May 1967, Australians voted overwhelmingly that the Australian Constitution be changed to be inclusive of Aboriginal and Torres Strait Islander people in Australian society. These changes enabled Aboriginal and Torres Strait Islander people to be counted in Australia's population and gave the Commonwealth government the power to make laws for Indigenous people concurrently with state governments. This referendum is often represented as having finally given Australia's Aboriginal and Torres Strait Islander peoples full citizenship.

However, as Michael Dodson, chair of the Australian Institute of Aboriginal and Torres Strait Islander Studies (AIATSIS), said recently in an address to traditional land-owners and native title-holders:

It is 40 years since the referendum where the Australian people decided to include us in the census, so we were no longer part of the flora and fauna, and to empower the Commonwealth to make laws on our behalf. I think that the referendum was a symbol of hope that finally the Government might use its powers to protect and support Aboriginal and Torres Strait Islander people, but apart from the *Land Rights Act* of 1976, there is little evidence that the state has the capacity to support our aspirations, let alone recognise and respect our sovereign status (Dodson 2007, p. 5).

In reality, citizenship has required Indigenous individuals to accept, reject or modify certain social models of 'independence', 'self-sufficiency', 'responsibility', and 'supervised modernisation' (Rowse 1998, p. 4). In this way, the settler society has, since the earliest decades of colonisation, ignored the existence of Indigenous societies or of Indigenous citizenship, which provided and continues to provide the first locus of social membership and identity for most Aboriginal and Torres Strait Islander people (Rowse 1998, p. 4).

Even after fully recognising Indigenous people in the Constitution, the government perpetuated the idea of Aboriginal people and Torres Strait Islanders as 'different' and 'other', all the while pursuing inclusion and the requirement to participate in structures and societies not of their own making. From this position, it is a logical step to define the health characteristics necessary for Indigenous people to belong, yet not be allowing them to belong completely. While ecological and environmental concerns are dealt with differently by Indigenous peoples in rural, remote and urban settings, the political goal of Indigenous people across the country is the same: Indigenous people want to be recognised and respected for their unique contributions to Australian society at the same time as participating in the mainstream of Australia's economic and social life. Since 2005, policy rhetoric has been to make Aboriginal people the same as the colonisers (Arabena 2005). Governments have been focused on integration: Indigenous people are to get the same opportunities and the same education that all Australians have in the hope that this makes Indigenous people the same. This policy framework has shifted considerably in recent times.

Two years on, in 2007, Commonwealth Indigenous policy shifted to ensure Aboriginal and Torres Strait Islander people demonstrate a level of competence and capacity in order to be admitted into mainstream society. New criteria are emerging to determine whether Indigenous people are good parents or whether they want to have good health. Indeed, these can seem to be the only things that are desirable. It has been argued by Indigenous academics and social commentators that such a viewpoint drove the Howard government to invoke its emergency powers for the land, health, welfare and military interventions in the Northern Territory that commenced in mid-2007. Given the amount of resources dedicated to saving vulnerable children from their incompetent parents, these interventions have variously been described as racist, oppressive and as a form of coercive reconciliation that is unprecedented in recent history.

In summary, the western health desiderata can be seen as largely constructed by non-Aboriginal others. Colonial regimes describe what kind of health Aboriginal people have and should have. As a form of resistance within identity politics, Aboriginal activists contrast this with ideas about the kind of health Aboriginal and Torres Strait Islander people have traditionally maintained, which is necessarily holistic, ecological and inclusive. These definitions of health have some similarities, but cannot effectively be meshed together. Indigenous peoples and public policy formulators are polarised by their views.

Indigenous world views assert that human health should not be placed above the health of everything around us in the environment. Indigenous people in many countries emphasise self-perceptions based on spirituality, tradition and sharing as oppositional to western rationalities. These identities have been strengthened and nourished through re-establishing and strengthening symbolic and practical connections between people, land and sea, and connections between ancient pasts and the present.

The inherent earth-caring philosophy of indigenous peoples is often challenged by governments, policy-makers and people who consider themselves to be members of mainstream society. Custodianship as a function of indigenous societies has been eroded by the imposition of Anglo-European socio-material systems on Aboriginal and Torres Strait Islander socio-material systems. This imposition is an infringement of the principle that certain peoples are fully intimate with certain lands and seas, and it is from these people we must learn to survive, thrive and flourish (Deloria 1968, p. 177). It is difficult to recognise the importance of indigenous philosophies and ecological knowledges when these have been marginalised in a globalised modernity. Despite this, Aboriginal and Torres Strait Islander people commonly view health in the context of the ecosystems with which they are intimate, a health and well-being that reflects membership in tribal and collective relationships with one another, the land and the environment (Sissons 2005).

At the start of the twenty-first century, when ecological degradation is of primary concern for governments and private enterprise around the globe, perhaps the challenge is the widespread adoption of an Indigenous ecological view—one which, when practised, has sustained ecosystems across the continent for 40 000 years. Aboriginal and Torres Strait Islander people had good health when contextualised as an interdependent part of an ecosystem, and suffer poor health in a society premised on global economic practices that degrade entire planetary processes which support complex life, including that of human beings. In future, taking a non-modern approach to issues of modernity, it may well be inconceivable to consider human health as separate from the environments in which we live.

Judged on outcomes, Australian governments—state and federal—have continually struggled to create good policy for Indigenous health. In any policy's implementation, the complexities in social, political and under-resourced settings have a major impact, so that the result is usually significantly different from its original objectives. For Indigenous peoples, the holistic health concept has best been incorporated at a regional level where collaborations between health, land, housing, environmental and funding bodies have seen effective implementation of these interrelated programs. However, on their own they too seem incapable of achieving sufficient improvements in Indigenous peoples' health.

A different view of health is required from policy formulation to im-plementation. It may be possible that, in between the universalist and holistic approaches, there exists a series of concepts that have not been recognised by either group. In this space between our different ways of thinking, there could yet emerge a shared understanding, a recognition of the ways in which we are all the same, where we can respect the differ-ences in our various ways of living well and being well.

Such a conceptual space, which some theorists are calling a 'third space', would have a relationship to physical space, to place. The nomadic culture of Aboriginal tribes was so foreign to the British colonisers that they did not recognise it. They invoked the designation of *terra nullius*—empty land, unoccupied—to justify their occupation. Many Indigenous people have stated that their actual being has been obliterated by the occupation. Thus the reclamation of space is necessary to overcome European occupation and the spatial technologies that were brought to take Australian places as their own (Muecke 2004, p. 14). It is important for Indigenous people to repossess the spatial sensitivities that overcome western notions of 'time' and the disrespectful inhabitation of Indigenous 'place'.

With some notable exceptions, health is yet to be conceived spatially. Yet human life is inherently spatial. This can be explored in relation to place, location, landscape, environment, home, city, region, territory and geography. Opening up such a conceptual space in Indigenous health policy would open the scope of, and the critical sensibility in relation to, already established spatial and geographic imaginations about where and how people live (Soya 1996, p. 1).

ART AND HEALTH

From the perspective of art history, the development over the last few decades of the Aboriginal art movement in central and northern Australia has been astonishing. In world terms, it is a brilliant efflorescence of artistic activity. Surprisingly, it has also been central to many discussions about Indigenous health and health care. We might suspect such a link from having identified the importance of freedom to health policy and a knowing that freedom of expression is a precondition for art. How does this work in practice? Pre-literate societies had a range of ways of communicating which are now encapsulated in artwork. These are a union bound by kinship and a profound knowledge of country, inspiring experimentation, evolution and freedom.

Arabena, who lived with the Pintubi people—many of whom are now exhibited in art galleries around the world—carries an enormous canvas around with her that she painted to facilitate discussions about risk behaviours leading to problems with reproductive health and a burden of sexually transmitted infections in Central Australia. A traditionally sensitive topic for open discussion, she found art a very powerful medium for engaging people in health issues. Her workshops have resonated with people in the Cape York communities, New Caledonia, a number of Southeast Asian countries and in China. She uses the canvas to help illustrate her words when negotiating with communities about identifying risk behaviours and working with communities to develop strategies to overcome these risks. When faced with implementing a complex policy initiative in remote area communities with people for whom English is a second or third language, she trialled painting a canvas as a method to negotiate a population-based screening strategy to test for notifiable sexually transmitted diseases.

The painting shows people relating strongly to their country. Arabena says she holds it up at public forums and tells people 'this is what we are going to do'. Then she places it on the ground and starts talking about its story, which she says is about sexual and reproductive health. Within two minutes, her audience is engrossed. It's her way of getting people to share a learning experience which is familiar to the audience members, but not in a manner that allocates blame to anyone. It has been a vivid tool and is understood as much by the indigenous people of New Caledonia as by a diverse range of peoples in Australia.

With her audience, she workshops the development of symbols that communicate the 'lifeways' of people in the community, including depictions of life, death, sexual coupling, risky behaviours, travelling, safety and establishing who might be communicated with about sexual health problems. This occurs for two or three days before actually talking about sex. One of the most exquisite symbols about sexual coupling came out of an art workshop in New Caledonia, in which a sea cucumber was inserted in a giant clam. Such an image is local but transcultural and does not rely on anyone's skills in verbal communication, thus facilitating discussion about health without social constraint. She has travelled to communities with an array of health-promotion resources, but finds using these can sometimes restrict the discussions to behaviours that are non-local. With the painting in hand, combined with being prepared to sit down and converse over three or four days, and allocating resources to people to develop their own paintings, she has found communities develop the most amazing array of resources to use for their own purposes.

The paintings were immediately disseminated at the end of the workshops. Often, they ended up tucked under old women's arms who could then move around the community encouraging information-sharing and problem-solving among themselves. This approach to facilitating community development through art saw the generation of more than 100 art pieces that depicted risky sexual behaviour and problem-solving tasks. Stories about the paintings were told and attached to photographs of the paintings—another educative tool for use in a community setting. These processes, while implementing a policy framework determined outside of a community context, also provided a forum in which policy could be developed within the community. A particularly interesting series of paintings aided the development of policy for managing an HIV-positive infection in a remote area community, including issues about who needed to be told and how, and the role of Aboriginal health workers. Other sessions saw the development of peer-education paintings for young people. A 'daytime/night-time' painting was developed in which in one half of the painting was yellow and represented daytime, with everyone sitting around behaving themselves, and half of the painting was black and represented night-time, with everyone congregating around cartons of grog and going off and having sex together with all the associated risks. Put simply, through telling stories while painting, people were able to understand health experiences, the consequence of risky behaviour and how to reduce risk.

Art and its use for such purposes encourages communities to develop their own capacity to express to other health professionals and policy-makers what their desires and aspirations are, all the time working from within their own health culture and experience. The art becomes an aspirational tool that permits open and frank discussions about topics that have not easily been discussed. In many cases, health-related art workshops have proved liberating for some members of those communities.

Arabena's work with indigenous peoples in the Asia-Pacific region produced art that described how important health was for people in their communities. Through these processes, individuals and collectives were able to depict the kind of freedoms they wanted and the motivations for achieving health. These workshops also showed that the mechanisms of health and care did not need to be confined to a clinical experience in order to promote freedom.

The Aboriginal art movement in Australia promotes individual artists, provides economic development for the communities to which they belong, and assists in the maintenance of a rich cultural heritage. The Pintubi Homelands Health Service, however, has also been able to sell its artworks to raise funds for public health infrastructure. The utilisation of art in this way covered new ground, primarily because the Pintubi people were able to raise over a million dollars to implement the kind of health care that they wanted. Recognising the trouble caused when families were dislocated from country and kin, the Pintubi practised self-determination, selling their art to establish a renal dialysis service in the Western Desert. This enabled Pintubi people requiring dialysis to go back to country for significant periods of time, rather than staying in Alice Springs or Katherine. The Pintubi Health Service has continued to evolve its own policies and programs. They were fortunate to have eminent leaders like Smithy Zimmerman, a skilful negotiator who had a great love of and determination for his people. As a role model, he enhanced people's belief about what they deserved and the attitude necessary to see it achieved.

Art has similarly been used to target a wide range of diverse populations in many Indigenous health programs: from Streetwise comics to Condoman posters (an Aboriginal man in a rubber suit, styled on the Phantom comic strip hero), commissioned by the Redfern Aboriginal Medical Service in the late 1980s, to its use in the Loomah traditional lifestyle for health project in the West Kimberley (Clapham, O'Dea and Chenhall 2007).

A great deal of value is now placed on the use of art for health gain in Indigenous communities. Arabena says she developed her use of art in part out of a level of exasperation caused by not being able to communicate effectively with people in a way that was deep and meaningful. If an outsider (as Arabena was to the Pintubi people) goes to a community to talk about health, it is rarely helpful to impose clinical interventions without reference to the lived experience of people in those places. Health workers in these settings needed to be able to find shared points of interest through open negotiation. If professionals are allowed the freedom to use their own creativity to develop their relationships with the community, they can achieve results unlike anything that might come from following a standard approach.

For health professionals and policy negotiators—Indigenous or not—deploying their creativity allows them to describe their own concerns and home truths. Sharing these truths creates trust. But while this can create breakthroughs in communication, the outsider also needs to be prepared to accept that Indigenous people are also free to choose not to talk or participate in what is being proposed. Open, shared communication strategies have the potential to be misused. For instance, some health research in Indigenous communities has resulted in betrayal of those individuals whose lives were significantly affected by the results.

True community control and self-determination require that discussions be open debates, that individuals can choose not to participate, and that if they do, they can recognise a shared benefit in participating. In this way, we can promote health beyond its specifically western construct, allowing people to engage in and disengage from such discussion, and take the conversation towards their own concerns and truths.

FROM SOCIAL DETERMINANTS TO DETERMINATION FOR BETTER HEALTH

In a liberal democratic society that espouses personal freedoms, people are free to choose their health behaviour, even if taxpayers may ultimately bear the cost of unhealthy behaviours. There is a tendency, however, for health professionals and politicians to insist that all people—including Indigenous people—should *want* better health. Within this modality, health interventions cannot be separated from a certain kind of morality, in which it is right for children to get immunised, for people to stop smoking and reduce their sugar intake, and so on. Around the world, moral codes signal the desired health behaviours and the desired health outcomes. To not want health in this way makes people undesirable, and in a way immoral. There is a particular history of aiming such messages at the most disadvantaged groups in society, reinforcing their undesirability at the same time as establishing criteria for moral superiority. In Australia, these messages have been a key feature of health service delivery for the Indigenous population. Health policy-makers need to recognise the consequences of ill-disguised paternalistic approaches.

A health transition is now occurring for Australia's Aboriginal and Torres Strait Islander population, some half a century after the same transition occurred for non-Indigenous Australian populations. While the transition may happen more or less quickly, it will result in longer adult life, with better health for Aboriginal people in the coming decades. The current demographics of Indigenous Australians show that, compared with the general population, Indigenous people have a much higher fertility rate, higher death rates, shorter life expectancy, much younger age structure and, as a proportion of the population, are growing faster (e.g. see Freebairn 2007). Half the Indigenous population is under the age of fifteen. The population health policy challenge is to facilitate a demographic transition towards longer life expectancy and lower death rates at all ages, particularly through the provision of better health care.

Such a transition will also require a cultural and social transition to reduce racism, improve education, alleviate poverty and create wealth. These are widely known as social determinants of health, a concept developed by Michael Marmot and colleagues (Marmot 2004). Marmot is a doctor who trained in Sydney and has gone on to become one of the world's most eminent epidemiologists. His analytical concept, and its mobilisation in the landmark report for WHO (Wilkinson and Marmot 2003), has had an enormous impact on health promotion policy at the highest level. Social determinants have captured the imagination of policy developers in Australia, becoming some of the most influential ideas in the governmentality of Indigenous health policy in that there are now new drivers of health policy which are more readily associated with the holistic health concepts espoused by Indigenous peoples. However, if not implemented with care, this concept can potentially underpin paternalism and fatalism.

Policy-makers routinely interpret data in a way that supports the kind of population health thinking they are used to. By understanding the social determinants of health, policy-makers have been able to focus health policy on things about society that affect health but are themselves outside the health sector as it is usually defined. These include things as diverse as education for girls and the importance (for reducing death rates) of collegiality in workplace relationships for middle managers. Marmot has explicitly identified being excluded from mainstream society as a key social determinant of the health of Indigenous people, stating that autonomy and social participation are so important for health that their lack leads to deterioration in health and well-being (Marmot 2004, p. 248). Yet knowledge about the known social determinants of health can make policy-makers feel it is pointless to consult. Why consult when these things are already determined? How does knowing the views of the people, whose health is inexorably determined, change anything?

However, while the causes of ill-health are frequently socially determined, the cures are not. Social interventions in particular, by the very fact that they are social, are mediated by dialogue and understanding. The success of interventions rests on the interplay between resistance, argument and cooperation. Metaphors of causal determinism are not helpful in understanding the dynamics of such interventions. Determination, on the other hand, is needed in spades.

To avoid paternalism for populations of people in the process of making an inter-generational health transition, policy-makers need to listen to the aspirations of the people for whom they are making policy. Listening to aspirations and taking account of these in policy work give people an opportunity to influence the direction of policy, and give the policy—when formed—a greater possibility of being relevant and effective. Effectiveness requires cooperation from the people affected by the policy. Even more importantly, it creates determination.

On the other side of paternalism in the mentality of Indigenous policy-making is the sense of fatalism that nothing has worked and that it is implausible to expect a positive impact from a planned intervention. There are some health professionals who have tried very long and hard through very good evidence-based population health strategies, using both personal and professional resources, to try to help Indigenous people, but have had no real effect. People have become resigned to their lot. Such fatalism emerges in communities faced with multiple chronic issues and social problems. They feel overburdened and downtrodden, and are unwilling to invest the personal energy necessary to change things.

Historically, social thinkers and visionaries have sought to recreate alternative spaces for more humane social orders, both within systems founded on the principles of western modernity (for example, socialist utopia movements within western democracies) and at other times by replacing these systems with entirely new social formations (for example, socialist countries). The purpose of this chapter is not to suggest how the current state of modernity in Australia might be restructured to accommodate Indigenous life in a more meaningful manner. What might be considered, though, is an attempt to conceive knowledge for the future outside of the constructs of western modernity.

For example, ecologists say that recognition of the universe as the primary is necessary for the earth's survival, particularly in any discussions of human affairs:

> Obviously the universe, the solar system and the planet Earth are the primary . . . We have no immediate access to anything intellectually or physically prior to or beyond the universe. The universe is its own evidence since there is no further context in the phenomenal world for explaining the universe. Every particular mode of being in the phenomenal order is universe-referent . . . The universe, in the phenomenal world, is the primary value, the primary source of existence, the primary destiny of whatever exists (Berry 1999, p. 190).

Placing the universe as the 'primary' might remedy the thoughts and actions that made human societies as independent as possible from the natural world and move away from 'human-centric' to 'universe-referent' modes of being.

Establishing the universe as the 'primary' enhances the capacity for people to move outside of western constructs of colonialism and establish ways and means for peaceful coexistence, superseding current policy agendas in which Aboriginal and Torres Strait Islander people are reconciled, educated and asked to participate in social structures alien to their own. For instance, Taiaiake Alfred, in his book *Wasase*, argues that a holistic view of the universe is an essential requirement for peaceful coexistence:

Without the recognition of the holism of the Universe, there can never be peace among peoples here on earth . . . Existing outside of Empire, Indigenous spiritualities can be the foundations for the cultures of universal responsibility and respect that are needed to achieve peaceful coexistence and ensure our survival on this earth (Alfred 2005, p. 266).

These knowledges distinguish the human species from all others, just as the human presence on earth distinguishes the ecology of our planet from other places in the known universe. In this way, we are all indigenous to this earth, and this universe. This is the truth of humanity. To know ourselves in this way, we will need many commentators who can attest to this fact. The Canadian intellectual John Ralston Saul, noting what was being said by Taiaiake, argues that the animist spirituality of many indigenous peoples, with its recognition of the networks of commonality between people, other living things and the world around us, offers an ethos that can help convey these truths. Saul has pointed out: 'We're seeing the return of aboriginals to a central role in Canada, the central role which they were guaranteed at the beginning . . . that return may be the thing that will save Canada as a civilization' (Saul 2005, p. 7).

While such things reflect the dislocation and despair that people are feeling inside Aboriginal and Torres Strait Islander communities, there do not appear to be any real opportunities to find lasting happiness in mainstream society either. Amidst the satisfaction people feel with their material progress, Robert Lane identifies a spirit of unhappiness and depression haunting advanced market democracies throughout the world, a spirit that 'mocks the idea that markets maximise well-being and the eighteenth century promise of a right to the pursuit of happiness under benign governments of people's own choosing' (Lane 2000, p. 1). Care must be taken when working with people to construct aspirations and build imagined futures in any community; there are many unhelpful myths that pervade ideals of happiness. This is doubly so for people who not only have trouble envisaging a better future, but who cannot envisage any kind of future at all. Without some cohesive idea about what happiness might be and whether its pursuit is worthwhile, the question of 'What is health?' has a certain hollowness, with the result that the basis of health remains elusive.

We in Australia all have our residence on this continent in common, and a cosmopolitan perspective can lift our discussions out of nationalist politics with its colonialist structures. The conception of Medicare as a universal health system, open to all Australians, to refugees and even to tourists whose countries offer a reciprocal arrangement, embodies this thinking to some extent. But it sets up the policy challenge of how Aboriginals and Torres Strait Islanders, as citizens and participants in government, and in consultation with other experts and government operatives, can make a health system that aspires to be universal and comprehensive work in complex settings to deliver the necessary health services wherever Indigenous people live.

The same challenges could extend in the near future to other indigenous people in the Pacific region. Around the world, global warming and civil conflict will drive large-scale population movements which liberal democratic countries will need to acknowledge and to which they will need to respond. Australia cannot isolate itself from the need to offer protection to people who face annihilation from ecological, political and other catastrophes. This could amount to several hundred thousand people who will want to enter Australia and retain their participation in a communal society.

For example, at a meeting of South Pacific governments, a range of leaders from island countries spoke of wide-ranging population displacement due to ecological changes, particularly rising sea levels and an increase in high-intensity weather events. The people of the Carteret Islands, a low-lying coral atoll and a part of Papua New Guinea, about 85 kilometres northeast of Bougainville, are the world's first global warming refugees; their islands are going under water and the population is being relocated to Bougainville. These refugees will need to seek new ways of living and aim to maintain their culture and communal existence.

Another Pacific island, Kiribati, has an exploitative colonial past. It has suffered through nuclear tests conducted on Kiribati's largest island by Australia's nuclear allies in the 1960s, and had its highest island extensively mined for phosphate, sold to farmers in Australia and elsewhere. Resettlements to the Solomon Islands and Fiji have already occurred.

In the last few years, the Australian government has had resettlement negotiations with Kiribati, which will be inundated as sea levels rise. Yet the Australian government has indicated that it will only accept them as individuals. Hopefully, common sense will prevail and we will recognise the value of assisting the immigration of a cohesive cultural group and recognise the resettlement as an event of two-way value, not patronise it as an act of charity to desperate people from a failed colony.

Understanding ourselves in the context of the coherency of the universe overrides the dominant geopolitical perspectives (states, nations, territories, globe) and provides a view of the world that could mark society and social policy in the years to come (Laszlo 2004, p. 80). This is not just a matter for analytical reflection. The mentality taken in the government's involvement in the geopolitics of climate change can have a profound effect on many people's lives over the coming decades.

Perhaps we need to consider the broad shape of a post-colonial society, and the way it deals not only with its citizens but its depleted natural surroundings. It is important to be mindful that there is no single enemy against which we are fighting. Rather, there is a disparate set of struggles, each of which will need to be addressed in its own peculiarity. This is the behaviour that gets things done, provided the activists channel their dissent in positive ways. We can take heart from national heroes like Vincent Lingari, who led the Gurindji people in the Northern Territory in a strike against the British beef baron Lord Vesty 40 years ago. Initially a strike for better pay and conditions, it became a cause that was taken up around the country, growing into a fight for land rights that culminated ten years later in the *Aboriginal Land Rights Act*. Tales of lesser heroism occur every day, such as when people conquer things in themselves and become better for it. There is heroism in the many men and women who have overcome their alcoholism, or a tendency to violence, or who have thrown off their own poverty. Such activism—personal, local and national—inspires others to do and be their best.

While a true belief in a worthy cause is wonderful, it is not enough. The activist has to be able to make things happen, which is where the politicking comes in for those who are funded by, but not under the control of, the bureaucracy. For the supportive activist within the bureaucracy, there is a need for pragmatism. It can be very hard work, with a need to deal with dissent and divisiveness and with the business interests that loom into the mix of governmental politics and community politics. But the need for negotiation also brings people together, and a shared collegiality can achieve a result.

9.

HEALTH PROTECTION

Crowding people together is inherently unhealthy. It allows diseases to spread between them, it allows violence to erupt between them, and it brings them together to increase the mortality from storms, earthquakes or fires. Urban living separates people from their water supply and makes the issue of sewerage and waste disposal a problem not just for themselves, but for their neighbours. Food supply can also present difficulties. The very fact of being together can also make a population an easier target for their enemies.

Nevertheless, population pressures have led to the rise and rise of urban living in the great cities of the world, and much of public health has developed as efforts to counter what has been called the urban penalty (e.g. see McMichael 2006). Urban societies have developed a range of public health technologies to ease the way of life and improve the healthiness of living in cities. Water and sewerage reticulation, food handling, vaccination, disease notification, outbreak identification and disease-control measures all play an important part in improving the health of urban populations.

Health systems, primarily oriented to contribute to social security within the state, also have an important relation to security from external threats. Historically, this included the assurance of a healthy enough population to stock the military as well as the provision of health care to people injured by war, other organised violence and natural calamities. Emergency planning against human and natural disasters is an important part of the civil defence of cities. Public health efforts also play their part in detecting and responding to terrorism. More recently, there has been a merging of communicable disease control strategies and emergency planning strategies in developing responses to expected epidemics such as pandemic influenza.

These technologies of disease control and population protection have become as complex and sophisticated as organ transplants and cancer treatment have in the clinical field. Clinical technology derives its power from molecular science and the know-how for the manipulation of bodily tissues. While these are important for health protection, the real power of public health actions derives from their connection to political power. Without this connection, a community's capacity to organise the protection of its health at a population level would be extremely limited. This connection to the power of the state is illustrated by the way communities organise for the safety of their water and food, protect against contagion and prepare to face disasters.

WATER SECURITY

Water and sewerage—access to clean water and disposal of human waste—have been central to human health since before urbanisation. Clean, clear running water from streams near their source has been recognised as healthful since ancient times. Conversely, the ancients warned to stay away from stagnant or odorous bodies of water. One problem with stagnant water is that it does not carry waste away. The simple logic of camping by a stream shows the principle of separation of drinking water from wastewater.

With the development of urban settlements of some size came the principle of reticulation, where water was piped in from clean sources for use and piped out in separate channels to dispose of wastewater. The aqueducts of ancient Rome and the infrastructure of many other ancient and medieval cities show the engineering solutions used to achieve reticulation of the water supply and sewerage. In the contemporary world, there is a key public health collaboration between the water utilities and public health officials in the provision and regulation of reticulated water supply and sewage disposal. In Australia, the National Health and Medical Research Council publishes guidelines for water quality that form the basis of quality control and regulatory systems in all states and territories for drinking water supply.

Population expansion, increasing use per head of water, increased agricultural use of water and the droughts that have affected Australia this century have led to a wide range of new water infrastructure projects being planned and implemented. The technology available for this current infrastructure activity is much more extensive than in the post Second World War period, when much of Australia's older water infrastructure was built. This new technology, including ultraviolet treatment and membrane filtration, is allowing desalination of sea water and water recycling from sewers and storm drains to drinking water in a planned and controlled way.

These projects have the potential to revolutionise the reticulation systems of contemporary communities. The planning and implementation are based on a close collaboration between public health authorities and water utilities. The public health issues brought up by recycling of drinking water in cities are perhaps the most complex problems in this field, and form the focus of the discussion below.

Much of the quality of recycled water depends not just on the engineering infrastructure, but on the systems of surveillance, monitoring and response in the regulatory framework that enable a more fine-grained oversight of the quality of water than earlier regulatory schemes allowed. These new regulatory schemes are set out in the National Health and Medical Research Council Drinking Water Guidelines' (2004) approach to risk assessment and risk management.

Achieving and maintaining water security is fundamental to the sustainability of any city. Quantity, quality, distribution, collection, treatment and public confidence are entwined to establish the security of water as a public good. It requires well-understood sources of water, sufficient storage to ride out expected variations in climate, high-quality treatment plants, a sound distribution network, separate collection and treatment systems for used water and stormwater, flexibility in the system and its components, extensive quality control across the system, and public confidence in the quality of water supplied.

In the grip of the prolonged drought in the first decade of the twenty-first century, Australian cities introduced an impressive range of water security measures. These included subsidies for more efficient household water use, price increases, major upgrades of water treatment plants, imposition of outdoor water use restrictions, supply of treated stormwater and wastewater for irrigation of parks, bringing old dams back on line, linking storage dams to maximise catchment potential, and extraction of water from unexploited water sources, including streams and aquifers.

Downstream reuse of wastewater is common around the world in river communities. Wastewater treatment plant outflows go into rivers. Towns downstream—like London on the Thames, or Jugiong on the Murrumbidgee—take up the river water, treat it and supply it for drinking. The process will typically be repeated several times over the course of the river. Time over the river course allows sunlight and the river ecosystem to digest any treatment by-products, organic chemicals or microbes that the outflow may contain.

Historically, however, recycling within a town has been avoided as part of the separation of the distribution of drinking water and the collection of used water, and this approach has been seen as fundamental to securing the quality of the drinking water supply. With the availability of new technology and advanced water systems engineering, things are changing. A number of cities around the world—including Singapore, Brisbane, London and San Diego—have recognised that controlled recycling can significantly improve water security.

Flanders in Belgium and Orange County in the United States take wastewater treatment plant outflows, treat the water again—including pushing it through a polyamide membrane—then put the treated water into the ground and take it out again through bores. Singapore pipes similarly treated water into its main reservoir. Queensland has commenced construction of a similar membrane treatment/pipe-to-reservoir scheme.

The drought in the first few years of the twenty-first century has been no worse, at least in the Canberra region, than the previous drought at the beginning of the twentieth century. However, rainfall in southeastern Australia is expected to decrease over the coming decades, and our population will grow—as will our water use.

In general, sewage outfalls amount to around half of the water supplied to a city. It is usually a steady, reliable water source. The quality of the outfall from large contemporary sewage treatment plants is pretty good. It is at least as good as the water in rivers flowing through farmland, better when stormwater runoff is flowing.

A water recycling system applied to the outfall can recycle around 60 per cent of the outfall. Allowing for some loss, it is now quite feasible to recycle 25 per cent of the water supplied to a city, and reduce the city's net water use from the environment by 25 per cent. This also improves the storage-to-use ratio of the existing dams. With this net water use reduction, a recycling scheme can provide greatly improved water security for a city, significantly reduce the likelihood of water restrictions being needed in the future, and greatly reduce the chance of the existing dams running empty. Combined with synergistic water infrastructure developments, it can allow a major expansion of the population.

The standard of treatment for recycling should be higher than the standard for downstream reuse of potable water because the cycling of the water can allow the build-up of contaminants generated within the cycle, creating the possibility that the concentration of a chemical or virus in the water may build up over months or years as the water cycles around.

This type of planned water recycling needs to be carefully designed and operated, through the whole cycle from drain to tap. Public flushing of drugs down the toilet should be discouraged. Industrial, hospital and laboratory waste discharge into the sewers needs to be closely controlled. Operation of the wastewater treatment plant must be optimised and kept under close surveillance, with careful monitoring of the outflow water. Careful consideration needs to be given to the potential for treatment to actually create contaminants—for example, chlorination acting on chemicals in the wastewater can create trihalomethanes (THM) and N-nitrosodimethylamine (NDMA), which can cause cancer in humans. If these are created, they need to be removed.

The conventionally treated water should then go through the best treatment process available to remove parasites, bacteria, viruses, organic molecules including pesticides, pharmaceuticals and hormones, and inorganic molecules including heavy metals and disinfection by-products.

Internationally, there is a consensus that the best available water treatment processes include reverse osmosis through a polyamide membrane. Imagine a semi-permeable membrane with pure water on one side and salty water on the other. Osmosis is the process whereby some of the pure water flows through the membrane to dilute the salty water. When pressure is applied to the salty water, the water flows in the reverse direction, increasing the volume of pure water and leaving more concentrated salty water behind. This process is called reverse osmosis.

The outflow from a conventional sewage treatment plant includes a significant load of very fine solids. If unfiltered, this water will block the reverse osmosis membranes, so it needs to be put through a microfiltration membrane prior to going through the reverse osmosis membrane. If the water is to be recycled with only a short transit time in the environment, it should then be put through an oxygenation step, including irradiation with ultraviolet light to degrade small molecules that can pass through the reverse osmosis membrane.

It is then beneficial for the clean water to flow through an aquifer if available, a wetland (natural or artificial) or a creek before reaching the storage. This allows some time in the environment (which becomes time to implement a response in the event a problem with the system is detected) and further adsorption or degradation of small organic molecules by soil organisms and plant root systems. Flow down a creek allows volatile molecules to escape into the air. Ideally, the storage should be large enough to provide an additional barrier that takes the treated water a few days to traverse before being drawn upon again. It should then go through a further conventional treatment plant before being supplied to the town.

The control of the recycling processes needs to be detailed and robust. It should include licensing conditions imposed by environmental and health regulators. It must aim for compliance with the National Drinking Water Guidelines. Treatment plants should be accredited. There needs to be an extensive sampling regime at critical control points in every step of the system, and regular testing for a wide range of microbes, unwanted molecules and physical properties such as water pressure and conductivity.

Plans must be in place for what to do when problems are detected. Staff must be trained and kept up to date, and teamwork needs to be encouraged between people with all the different roles involved. Regular reports must be provided to the regulators, government and the public. Problems should be disclosed and dealt with openly as they arise.

A number of factors are at play that will increase the pressure for Australian cities to adopt water recycling. Population growth, our generally arid climate and expected declines in rainfall are the sticks. Improving technology, growing international experience and reducing membrane costs are the carrots.

Recycling plants and dams are expensive. They are major pieces of infrastructure for the sustainable development of any city and their cost is comparable to a multi-storey office block or a section of new dual-carriageway road. International experience shows that water recycling is often the most cost-effective way to bring on a new source of water in areas where water is scarce, compared with new dams, pipeline projects or desalination plants.

The impact of the recycling on the environment should be positive or neutral rather than negative. By-products of the treatment process, such as sludge, salt and wastewater, should be disposed of without negative environmental impact. The whole process should not result in net carbon dioxide release into the atmosphere. Clean energy should be sourced for the process or carbon sinks established as part of the set-up.

Recycling is complex. The design, research and development of the process should not be rushed. The different components need to be tested thoroughly and commissioned in the proper sequence. The water should not be drawn upon until everything is working smoothly, all monitoring systems are in place and the quality of the water has been proven.

Citywide recycling will be much cheaper than widespread adoption of residential greywater recycling and installation of rainwater tanks to reduce demand for town water. Of course, the two approaches can go hand in hand, and motivated householders who take care to follow rainwater and greywater reuse guidelines are making an important contribution to reducing our demand for water.

However, a 25 per cent reduction in demand through onsite residential measures would be extremely difficult to achieve. Large sticks and large carrots would be required. Making a myriad of unmotivated householders responsible for the maintenance and use of the systems could create multiple small health hazards that cannot effectively be regulated. Systems of self-reliance need much more land and space between neighbours than the quarter-acre block provides. Urban living requires a collective approach to natural resource use and waste disposal, and water is no exception.

FOOD-BORNE DISEASE AND COMMUNICABLE DISEASE CONTROL

As with water, public health professionals have a keen interest in assuring that the food supply does not cause disease. This is reflected in the public health field's professional and statutory interests in the primary production of food, the processing of foodstuffs, the logistics of transporting and supplying food, and in its preparation and serving as meals.

The microbiological basis of disease prevention through food handling is well understood. However, improvements continue to be made in detection and detailed typing of micro-organisms involved in food-borne disease outbreaks. Syndromic surveillance of gastroenteritis presentations in emergency departments is able to detect food-borne disease outbreaks more readily than serendipitous medical reporting of linked cases of gastroenteritis. The Oz Food Network in Australia and emergency department syndrome surveillance systems such as the AEGIS system in Boston are allowing public health action to be taken to control gastro-enteritis outbreaks where previously these may have gone undetected.

An interesting dynamic in food handling from the public health point of view is the public health benefit of providing less-processed food directly to consumers. Minimum processing improves food's nutritional value and energy balance because processing often drives up energy density, which refers to vitamins, saturates and fat in processed food. However, unprocessed food does not keep so well and is more prone to contami-nation with pathogenic micro-organisms. The more detailed application of public health principles in food handling, and the greater capacity of public health surveillance to detect problems and to regulate the food industry are assisting in the logistics of distributing less-processed food from producer to consumer. This can be seen in the flourishing of sushi restaurants and the expansion of seafood distribution networks through to the increased floor space devoted to fresh fruit and vegetables in our supermarkets.

It is worth remembering that as recently as my parents' generation, many children in the western world grew up knowing hunger. My father used to call it 'special sauce' that made all food delicious in his large family in pre-war Manchester. Domestic food rations during the Second World War actually led to an improvement in the diet and availability of food for many of the poor in the north of England.

In the postwar period, the food industry in the west largely overcame hunger, although this has come at a cost because providing highly processed, high-energy density, highly saturated fat-based food has produced a range of other health problems. Much of the policy being developed to tackle the recent problems of western obesity is based around shifting the processing and logistics of food towards a less transformed product being consumed. This is being made possible by improved food technology, along with the improved technologies of public health in the regulation and surveillance of and response to food-borne disease problems. This can be seen in the recent addition to the Australia and New Zealand Food Standards of standards around food preparation in high-risk food businesses such as those in residential care facilities and hospitals. The susceptibility of consumers in these settings makes the nutritional content on the one hand, and the bacteriological purity on the other, especially important.

More direct technologies of communicable disease control include vaccination, surveillance through disease notification programs and outbreak-control efforts. Vaccination is one of the standard developments in public health, and indeed of modern science. The elimination of smallpox in the 1980s is perhaps the biggest single achievement of public health. The elimination of polio is tantalisingly close. Like the smallpox virus, the polio virus exists outside the laboratories only in its human hosts. At the time of writing, polio is endemic only in Nigeria and the Afghanistan–India–Pakistan border areas (visit www.polioeradication.org to see the current situation). Global eradication programs such as these are reliant not just on the availability of an effective vaccine, but also on population health technology to achieve sufficient coverage so that every last wild viral particle is eradicated from the planet. These population technologies are as complex and sophisticated as the molecular technologies of vaccine production.

Without detailed population programs, immunisation rates above 80 per cent of the total population are difficult to achieve. Australian immunisation policy in the last decade has been very successful in this regard, with the proportion of fully immunised children lifted from around two-thirds in the mid-1990s to between 90 and 95 per cent in 2006. Childhood immunisation rates had been in decline since the early 1980s. This worsened in the Medicare era with the transfer of responsibility for distribution of vaccines from the Commonwealth to the states in the 1988 Medicare agreements. In the mid-1990s, the Commonwealth, under health minister Michael Wooldrige, resumed lead responsibility for population vaccination rates. It implemented a range of general practice-based strategies together with the Australian Childhood Immunisation Register and requirements implemented with the help of state governments for parents to demonstrate full vaccination of children on commencement of school. Public opposition to such aggressive measures has turned out to be much lower than feared, with only 2 per cent of the population being objectors to vaccination on deliberate grounds. This has meant that, with strong encouragement but not compulsion, vaccination rates of 95 per cent have routinely been achieved. However, it is a matter of ongoing vigilance and energy to maintain rates close to that level.

A particular challenge for childhood immunisation has been the growing complexity of the schedule of vaccines recommended by the National Health and Medical Research Council. This has largely been technology driven, with the commercial release in the first few years of the twenty-first century of vaccines for meningococcal disease, chickenpox and human papilloma virus. The development of technologies that can combine vaccines into a single injection or to reduce the number of injections needed to achieve immunisation are important to pursue in order to achieve some simplification of the schedule.

Some of the difficulties here are illustrated by influenza. Influenza vaccination has serious limitations. It requires annual vaccination with a triple-antigen mix effective against the three most common circulating flu viruses of any given year. Because of the changes in which strains of influenza are circulating, the vaccine also needs to be changed. This produces difficulties for the acceptability and cost-effectiveness of influenza vaccination (Dugdale 2007). Repeat vaccination also causes a large number of adverse reactions, including local pain in more than 20 per cent of people and influenza-like symptoms lasting for a day or two in around 10 per cent of people. These problems combine to have made it unacceptable to include influenza in the national recommendations for universal childhood vaccination.

Let's turn now to when prevention hasn't worked. Economists talk about 'externalities' when your choices affect others. A particular externality for public health is what you do when you have a communicable disease. Because of your potential to pass on the infection to others, the decision to treat or not to treat affects not just yourself, but has an external impact on those around you. Public health authorities work with general practitioners, emergency departments and pathology laboratories to obtain notification of patients with communicable diseases of particular public health importance. These include readily treatable conditions like gonorrhea and syphilis; conditions less easy to treat, but where treatment still makes a significant difference, such as HIV, hepatitis C, hepatitis B and tuberculosis; conditions that can be passed on through the food and water supply, such as salmonella and epidemic gastroenteritis; exotic conditions that have not yet established a foothold in Australia, such as malaria and yellow fever; and diseases that have been eradicated from the planet but may return, including SARS and smallpox.

The Disease Notification System forms the backbone of the outbreak-identification efforts of communicable disease control teams in all states and territories. With appropriate surveillance, higher than background levels of specific diseases will be noticed. Reported cases may be linked by a common exposure or address. More recently, syndrome surveillance systems have been established which monitor symptoms being reported to emergency departments. Specific symptoms of interest include gastrointestinal and respiratory symptoms. Patterns of injuries may also be detected (for example, the outbreak of broken legs detected by the ACT's emergency department information systems due to people falling off their roofs as they tried to prepare their houses for the 2003 bushfires). Once a cluster of illnesses is identified, samples can be obtained, analysed or reanalysed to look for specific strains that may link cases. Such detailed surveillance then underpins the outbreak-control efforts which may include simple hygiene measures, effective treatment through antibiotics, quarantine or lesser forms of isolation, along with greater efforts for case-finding. For many conditions, there will also be efforts to identify the source of the outbreak and eliminate or mitigate it. Specific actions vary by disease, and range from vaccination programs to removal of foodstuffs from the supply chain, to control of mosquitos for vector-borne diseases such as malaria, to changing the source of the water supply or closing down sewage outflows.

Communicable disease outbreak identification and control technologies rely for their success on the sophisticated bringing together of many different parts of the health and urban infrastructure systems, timely communication and the following of detailed evidence-based protocols. Their success has made it more likely that respiratory and food-borne disease outbreaks in the community will be identified, which in turn has fuelled community expectations of a robust public health response to the identified outbreaks.

DISASTER RESPONSE

The key driver for emergency response planning is the natural disaster. Interestingly, these seem to be happening more frequently for any given scale of incident. This is in part because of world population growth and also because of climate change due to human activity. Extreme weather events have become more frequent and this is expected to continue. The population explosion on the Indian Ocean rim meant that the tsunami of 2004 killed many more people than the tsunami associated with the eruption of Krakatau in the 1890s.

In any sizable human population, emergencies happen every day. All medium-sized country towns and larger populations have emergency services: police, ambulance, fire brigade and a hospital with an emergency department, along with public health surveillance and response personnel. Together, these emergency services form the backbone of disaster response. In general, civil disaster response plans are designed to coordinate police, fire, ambulance, emergency department and public health authorities. In scenarios where local civil defence coordination will be insufficient, there are plans for calling on back-up from other jurisdictions and the armed forces. Sitting underneath these regional disaster plans are institutional disaster plans for health facilities, utilities (water, gas, electricity), residential care facilities and commercial buildings (all of which have fire and evacuation plans).

Underlying disaster response planning is the need for action in response to a disaster. If there is no planned and coordinated action, there will still be action. People involved or concerned with the disaster will do things in response to it. Disaster plans as preparation for coordinating the disaster response aim to harness this energy so that it can make a positive impact on the disaster and ameliorate its adverse effects. Sometimes the evidence we would like to drive the planning and response efforts does not exist, particularly in unique events. In these situations, the disaster response may be driven as much by the need to calm public anxiety and provide a framework for the actions of those in the scene as it is by sound evidence about what would produce the best impact in the situation. In this way, disaster response is a combination of evidence-based planned action together with an implementation of the managerial principles related to achieving large-scale coordinated action: strong leadership, promoting team spirit, efficient use of resources, a careful eye for morale, two-way communication up and down the chains of command, and positive recognition from up the chain about the efforts of those at the front line.

Disaster exercises do more than just test disaster plans. They also build team spirit and provide people with the confidence to act in a co-ordinated way when faced with a real disaster. This includes confidence in knowing what to do, confidence in their superiors, and confidence in the plans themselves.

Disaster planning encompasses prevention, mitigation, response and recovery. Disaster exercises typically focus on the response component of these plans, including asset mobilisation, triage, command and control chain testing, and the involvement of volunteers. More recently, the exercises have also focused on actually commencing the disaster response—that is, moving from the surveillance phase of preparation to the response phase—and also the commencement of recovery, especially recovery planning and commencement of recovery asset mobilisation. There has also been a resurgence of interest in simple drills testing a very limited component of a disaster plan: building evacuation; drug mobilisation for prophylaxis of front-line personnel in disease outbreak disasters; and rolling out assets such as decontamination shower sets, heavy machinery and field treatment facilities. During the current century, the increased involvement of the Commonwealth in disaster response has led to a number of exercises emphasising the testing of command and coordination mechanisms between jurisdictions. This national government interest has been driven by the fear of an information technology malfunction at the turn of the millennium (Y2K), the terrorist attacks on New York's World Trade Center and the Pentagon in 2001 (9/11), and the avian flu outbreak leading to fear of a human influenza pandemic of the H5N1 influenza strain. Against this backdrop, there have been a number of large-scale bushfires (such as that in the Australian Capital Territory in January 2003 where over 500 houses were burnt down), and the cyclones, storms and floods to which Australia is prone.

In the event of a disaster or related emergency, health systems can respond in a number of preplanned ways. The traditional governmentality of the emergency response draws on military models of command and control, in which available resources are commandeered from their routine operating environment and controlled through a hierarchy especially established to coordinate the response to the emergency.

Disaster preparedness involves planning at all levels of the health system—national, state and territory, area health service, hospital and other health services. We will now consider the features, strengths and weaknesses of these two styles of response.

The command response has its origins in the military style of administration. The definition of a disaster is usually given as a circumstance that overwhelms the normal operation of the agency, necessitating an extraordinary reorganisation of the resources controlled by the agency through the activation of the disaster plan. Response strategies are formulated at the top of the authority hierarchy in a command centre that ideally receives rich information about the disaster and the activities of agencies in the field. Directions are relayed down the lines of control, specified in the disaster response plan, to agencies or components of agencies that reassign the resources under their control to the disaster response.

More recently, a new mentality has been delineated in which standard lines of control are expected to drive a surge of capacity to handle the demands arising from the emergency. The surge response uses the ordinary channels of managerial control and the ordinary resources of an agency or set of agencies. The disaster is responded to with a short- to medium-term surge in activity, which may include staff being recalled from leave or being asked to work longer hours, or increased throughput and work rates, coupled with deferral of inessential tasks.

Contemporary emergency response planning requires both these modes of response to be available, depending on circumstances.

TERRORISM

Since medieval times when life could be summarised as nasty, brutish and short, modern society has become civilised through the development of shared norms abhorring murder, a distaste for violent assault and a willingness to accept moral responsibility for one's actions. Paradoxically, this has resulted in a concentration of the means of violence in the apparatus of state. At the same time, the deployment of state power has become less personal and more responsive to the requirements of the state itself. The use of violence by the state is not subject to moral calculation in the same way that the personal use of violence is. The policeman who takes the Aborigine to the gaol does so because the court has meted out a gaol sentence, not because the policeman's desire to capture and incarcerate another man is stronger than the guilt he feels about doing this. The civilised society is one in which violence has ceased to figure in the everyday life of its citizens. In part because of this, and in part because of the concentration of the means of violence in agencies of state that have been designed to operate in an impersonal manner, the civilising process actually increases the potential for larger scale and morally abhorrent state-controlled violence.

Medical science and health system design have long had a reciprocal relationship with violence in general and war in particular. In a sense, all warfare is biological. The siege of a walled city, leading to starvation and death of the inhabitants, was a mainstay of territorial battle tactics in ancient and medieval times and has remained common in modern warfare. The health of the English proletariat was brought into focus by reports concerned with their fitness to fight in the Boer War of the late nineteenth century. Surgical techniques developed rapidly in Napoleon's armies and during the first and second world wars of the twentieth century. The term 'Resident Medical Officers', used to describe the doctors who provide the mainstay of basic medical care in Australia's public hospitals, harks back to the military. The discovery and development of penicillin by Fleming and Florey gave the Allies a major advantage during the Second World War. An extension of the siege is the use of economic sanctions against whole countries by the United Nations, used most recently against Iraq between the 1991 Gulf War and the 2003 US-led war. The blockade extended to medical supplies (although not food), and was an important cause of the deaths of around half a million children in Iraq during those years (UNICEF 1999).

The relationship between health, health system development and violence is always historical and particular. In recent years, systems of surveillance and emergency response in Australia (and elsewhere) have evolved according to a biosecurity agenda concerned with terrorism linked to the military excursions of countries with a largely Christian population into countries with a largely Muslim population. Before discussing this evolution, it is worth considering the current historical context of violence at the international level.

John Keane, an Adelaide-educated, London-based academic, has provided a simple analysis that situates the major contemporary concerns in western democracies about national level and international violence within a triangle of types of violence. The first side of the triangle is the potential for 'nuclear-tipped' (Keane 2004, p. 22) military activities by the states with nuclear arms capability, many of which have engaged in military adventures over the last decade. This is a quite different nuclear scenario than was felt to be the main line of possibility in the Cold War between the two superpowers from the mid-1950s to the mid-1980s. While the threat of escalation of nuclear exchanges towards mutually assured destruction has receded substantially since that time, the possibility of some nuclear weapons use in the current period cannot be discounted. Keane notes that: 'The US State Department currently lists forty-four governments endowed with nuclear weapons capacity' (Keane 2004, p. 23).

The second side of the triangle is the 'violence unleashed in uncivil wars' (Keane 2004, p. 24) in isolated states where the majority of the population may become enmeshed in murder and atrocity. Examples include Sudan, Rwanda and Bosnia. Keane contrasts this with the traditional understanding of the civil war, where 'combatants were locked into a violent but disciplined struggle for control over the key resources of territorial state power'. However: 'Within uncivil war zones, violence becomes a grisly end in itself' (Keane 2004, p. 25).

The third side of the triangle is global terrorism as it is depicted in the War Against Terror being led by the United States, with activity dating perhaps from the early 1980s and including the Sarin gas attack in the Tokyo Metro in 1995, plane crashes into the World Trade Center and Pentagon in September 2001, and suicide bombers in Bali in 2002. This type of terrorism is different from terrorist activity by states against their own subjects, or guerrilla activity aimed at the occupation of territory, or classical terrorism aimed at securing a negotiation with a governmental enemy (Keane 2004, p. 27). The new 'apocalyptic terrorists thought of themselves as engaged in total war against an enemy that was unworthy of negotiation and incapable of compromise' (Keane 2004, p. 29). Keane quotes Habermas's insight that: 'The new terrorism we associate for the time being with the name "al-Qaeda" makes the identification of the opponent and any realistic assessment of the danger impossible. This intangibility is what lends terrorism a new quality' (Habermas et al. 2003, p. 29).

This depiction of a triangle of violence identifies three logically discrete types of violence of grave concern to the nation state, and also captures the current expression of public and polity concern about those matters. It allows us to see terrorism in its contemporary context. This is important because terrorism has become a new driver of public health surveillance reform and emergency response planning, and poses particular difficulty because of the impossibility of any realistic assessment of the danger.

The all-hazards approach taken to emergency planning in Australia makes no distinction between natural and social events. The passenger jet that runs off the runway, the train derailment, the bridge collapse, the dam burst are all well-recognised scenarios for exercises to test emergency plans, and all have occurred in reality in Australia, evoking actual emergency responses. Like natural disasters, there is no enemy, no person or group that has planned the episode, and so no need to consider the unfolding of the episode from the perpetrator's point of view.

Terrorist acts are designed to create terror at the time of the event, especially among the people immediately involved. However, unlike the French Terror of the early 1790s or the totalitarian regimes of Hitler or Stalin, where widespread violence cowed large parts of the population into a continuing state of terror, the threat of contemporary terrorism places susceptible members of the broad population into a state of anxiety rather than terror.

Anti-terrorist responses such as surveillance, body searches at airports, restriction of movement (e.g. across the grassed roof of Parliament House) and secret intelligence-gathering also generate widespread low-level anxiety, partly through these activities themselves and partly by amplifying the anxiety caused by terrorism itself. This is somewhat ironic, as the responses may actually be designed more to reduce anxiety than to ameliorate risk. A federal cabinet minister made this clear: 'To be tactful about these things, a lot of what we do is to make people feel better as opposed to actually achieve an outcome' (Vanstone 2005). Part of the reason for this disconnect is the lack of evidence about what works and what doesn't. Vanstone's remarks were made at a time when the Australian government was reviewing the ban on metal knives being provided with in-flight meals, at a time when wine glasses were still provided and, according to the minister, could be just as menacing: 'You just smash your wine glass and jump at someone, grab the top of their head and put it in their carotid artery and ask anything' (Vanstone 2005).

One approach to this problem has been to recognise the distinction between the motivation and the means for a terrorist attack. It might be more efficient to concentrate the surveillance effort on those motivated to execute an attack rather than to increase widespread surveillance of the means of an attack at possible sites such as airports, train stations and sports stadiums. Targeted surveillance of suspects requires intelligence, either through informants or infiltration of social networks of people who might have motivations to create terror. It also raises somewhat different civil liberties concerns than widespread low-level surveillance of the means for an attack.

Health system activities relating to terrorism occur in surveillance, analysis and response as part, or as an extension, of the relationships for disaster responses that the health sector has with other emergency and security agencies. Health laboratories—for example, those forming the Australian Public Health Laboratory Network—may be involved in analysis of 'white powder incidents' involving suspicious materials. This would usually be at the request of the police or fire brigade, and ideally would be carried out according to protocols agreed between police, fire brigade and health authorities for the handling and investigation of hazardous materials, or materials that might be hazardous.

Public health agencies may be involved in surveillance and analysis of symptom clusters that may be caused by substances released by terrorists. This is an extension of their normal role in population health surveillance. Treating clinicians already report a variety of notifiable diseases. The Australian Emergency Department Information System, installed in each emergency department around Australia, provides an important database to interrogate for symptom clusters. With expansion of information and communications technology for health, it has become possible to regularly sift data from these sources looking for patterns of interest, such as gastrointestinal symptoms compatible with widespread malicious poisoning from botulin toxin or ricin, or notifications of communicable diseases linked to biological warfare agents such as pulmonary anthrax or smallpox.

Health agencies may also be involved with police and national security agencies in the analysis of intelligence—for example, in advising on the plausibility of threats where expert medical knowledge can help separate real threats from pranks, or on the elaboration of realistic scenarios in the face of actual threats.

Once a deliberate act of terror has occurred that has caused, or could cause, human injury, health authorities will be involved in the response. This includes continuing surveillance and analysis of what has happened, and planning for what can be expected to happen. In the response to natural or accidental disasters, health authorities are central to the intelligence and analysis effort. Their value in this effort comes from their extensive field network of health personnel, their knowledge of the impact of various things and events on human health, and their inherent flexibility in responding to community demand for health services.

NEW INFECTIONS

Contemporary scientific methods provide a tremendous capacity for discovery and surveillance of things in the world that may affect human health. A number of communicable diseases appear to have arisen anew in the last few decades, at a time when this could be observed by the medical and public health world. Some of these have emerged in the midst of modern medical practice, including multi-resistant staphylococcus and multi-resistant tuberculosis. Others have emerged in the midst of large human populations by transfer from food source animals, including SARS, highly pathogenic avian influenza (H5N1) and ebola virus. Others appear to have emerged from wild animals, including HIV from chimpanzees. The identification of these diseases and the characterisation of the micro-biological agents that cause them have been among the most exciting efforts in modern science in the last few decades.

Acquired Immune Deficiency Syndrome (AIDS) was first reported as an epidemic disease in 1981, once it had caused a cluster of immuno-deficiency related pneumonia among gay men in Los Angeles (US CDC Morbidity and Mortality Weekly Report 18 June 1981), with the Human Immunodeficiency Virus (HIV) that causes AIDS identified in 1983 (Barre-Sinoussi et al. 1983). HIV/AIDS is now a major health problem around the world, with 40 million people living with HIV in 2006, including around 4 million people infected and 3 million people who died from AIDS in 2006. The Australian government updates its national HIV/AIDS strategy every three years, including substantial recurrent funding. The first strategy came out in 1989 (Commonwealth of Australia 1989), when it was the first major national response to a specific condition since the introduction of Medibank as a unified national health system.

Severe Acute Respiratory Syndrome (SARS) was first reported from Guangdong province to Chinese authorities in November 2002, and the coronavirus that causes SARS was identified at Hong Kong University in March 2003; a test for the virus had been created by the end of that month (Rizaz 2003). International efforts to control the SARS outbreak by iden-tifying and isolating cases were successful in breaking the chain of human-to-human transmission by July 2003. There have been three sub-sequent incidents where SARS was contracted from laboratory samples, and one incident in Guangdong where the virus was contracted from the community, presumably from animals. In this and the three laboratory incidents, cases were identified promptly and the chain of transmission quickly stopped in one to three generations of transmission (WHO 2004b). Clearly, the disease has the potential to re-emerge, and surveillance therefore continues. The WHO response to SARS was a magnificent example of the surge response to an international emergency. WHO worked with health professionals on case identification, worked with national authorities on epidemiological surveillance and analysis, and drew together an international network of laboratories for the identification of the virus and development of a reliable test for it. This response demonstrated the depth and sophistication of resources that were prepared to mobilise to tackle a new global outbreak—and therein lies an important part of the story about the world's actual capacity to cooperate in the face of a major new health threat.

The mid-2000s pandemic of influenza amongst birds resulted in human cases of infection with a novel form of Highly Pathogenic Avian Influenza A (HPAI H5N1) virus from October 2003 (WHO 2004a). The lethality of human infection with HPAI H5N1 is quite high at over 30 per cent of identified cases, but human-to-human transmission with this virus does not occur—at least not to any significant extent. However, there is widespread concern that the virus may mutate or that the genetic component of the HPAI H5N1 virus that makes it highly lethal in humans may be incorporated into another strain of influenza which is transmitted easily between humans. Either scenario could result in a pandemic amongst humans that kills millions of people.

HIV, HPAI H5N1 and SARS all developed in animals and then transferred into the human population. They join Lissa virus, Hanta virus, vCJD (mad cow disease), West Nile virus, Lyme disease and Q fever—to pick just a selection that have received sufficient policy attention to merit press coverage in Australia over the last decade—and the many other zoonoses, meaning that they infect animals and humans and that humans generally acquire their infection from an infected animal. Health system responses to zoonoses need to combine with responses from other sectors, in particular animal health authorities. Cooperation across human and animal health authorities has long been poorly coordinated; however, some commentators are optimistic that it has been improving in recent years, through sustained effort (Marano et al. 2005). This has been helped by joint disaster response exercises in Australia—for example, around foot and mouth disease in 2004 and HPAI H5N1 in 2006.

Pandemic influenza planning is a mixture of communicable disease control and emergency planning. These two fields have strong but quite separate intellectual traditions, both of which have been intensifying in recent years. Mixing them together for pandemic influenza planning has been quite complex and resource intensive across the health system and more broadly. The danger for developing policy in relation to pandemic influenza is that the historical lack of depth in the bringing together of disease control and emergency planning could result in what we might call 'push button policy', which addresses the lobbying matters and hot issues currently under discussion in the representative bodies involved in such policy development (e.g. concerning remuneration, research funding, professional development and working conditions). More than round-table conversation is required to achieve rational policy formation that can be expected to achieve better population outcomes in the event of a pandemic (e.g. see Phillips et al. 2007).

The clinically driven science behind these disease identification and response efforts is now extremely powerful, and to some extent almost routinised in its global coordination when a new cluster of symptoms appear that fit Koch's postulates, identifying them as caused by a trans-missible agent. In addition, the disease-control mechanisms useful for these new diseases still relate fundamentally to water and sewerage, food handling, vaccination, disease notification, outbreak notification and control coordination efforts, as discussed above. To adapt a phrase, the price of freedom from communicable disease is eternal vigilance. Just like freedom itself, freedom from communicable disease is never complete, and always rests on the willingness to struggle for it.

10.

HEALTH POLICY ACTIVISM

MANAGEMENT COMMITMENT

As a generalisation, people working in health policy and management are a very committed lot. The health field is attractive to people who are motivated to make a difference in society. It is also a field of old institutions and long traditions, so it can feel very conservative. This contributes to a sense among many health workers engaged in caring for patients that there is a lot that needs to be done in policy, and that management could do a lot better. Consequently, there is a large talent pool of people willing to put their mind to policy issues or who are willing to take on management responsibilities, despite the widespread poor regard in which managers and policy workers are held by clinicians at the coalface.

As managers and policy workers, it is important that we don't take our commitment for granted. It requires some reflection, both on its motivations and on its deployment. This chapter begins by analysing the interaction of public sector managers and consumer advocates. Taking the perspective of the manager, the analysis has a theoretical and a practical angle. First, a central theoretical debate is reviewed to provide a reference point from which to understand action taken by managers. Second, an analysis is developed of strategically important parts of the terrain of interaction between managers and advocates. This covers formal consumer consultation exercises and the usefulness of public policy skills.

It examines theoretical issues in the debate over the relation between the managerial values of efficiency and effectiveness, and program values of equity and access. If we accept the pervasiveness of managerial forms of organisation within the public service, I argue that the reconciliation of these values of efficiency, effectiveness, equity and access can be achieved by the new managers making a commitment to equity and consultation. The value of equity is closely related to the outcomes focus of program management within the welfare bureaucracy. Although this reconciliation sits fairly easily at the level of values, it is problematic and under-theorised at the level of practice. Scant reference to it can be found in managerialist texts.

This reconciliation calls for a review from the manager's perspective on the practical use of consumer consultation in public sector decision-making, and the issues involved in actually managing consumer consultation. This review concludes that, while various managerial techniques can facilitate such consultation, more traditional public service skills in the coordination of processes and in policy formulation also need to be deployed.

From time to time, a debate runs through the Australian *Journal of The Royal Australian Institute of Public Administration* about, on the one hand, the instrumental operation of the public service—with the emphasis on efficiency, effectiveness and letting the managers manage—and, on the other hand, the values of the public service—with the emphasis on fairness, access, equity and participation.

One side of this debate claims that public sector managerialism supports these values by providing the focus on outcomes necessary to actually achieve better access, greater equity and more participation in fields where this is an objective of the government. Michael Keating (1989) has articulated this viewpoint, stating that 'the pursuit of social justice has been significantly enhanced through the introduction of program management and budgeting and the better evaluation of programs which it has encouraged . . . the concern for effectiveness is also a concern for equity' (1989, p. 129).

On the other side of the debate, the economic rationalism found in managerialism and the particular management tools it has imported from the private sector are seen as actually undermining these public service values. Anna Yeatman (1990b) has summed this up as follows: 'In the current reconstitution of public bureaucracies to fit the economic rationalist model of government, the values of equity and access have been residualised . . . They have been abandoned along with the discourses of citizenship and public service' (1990b, p. 21).

As Yeatman points out, the concern for equity and participation cannot be subsumed under a concern for effectiveness, and is not a central concern of program management techniques. However, there is a sense in which Keating can be right, in that if equity and participation are a central concern of the manager, then program management can enhance the effective implementation of these concerns. If we accept this, the debate about whether managerialism in the Australian Public Service promotes or undermines the values of equity and access highlights the importance of a commitment on the part of management to the active participation of citizens in public service decision-making.

The focus on outcomes has drawn managers of welfare programs to evaluate the realities of working with their target groups and at least consider the value of consultation for effective program implementation. The two-way dependency between the public service and the public is expressed by Yeatman (1990a) in her discussion of citizen involvement in government policy formation: 'The citizenry also has a significant relationship to these policies once they have assumed the specific features of programs . . . Not only is their cooperation required—a passive sense of citizen participation—but as citizens demand more of government services these services become dependent on the active participation of citizens in order to have their demands reflected in the service' (1990a, p. 51).

The arguments against consumer consultation are a pervasive part of everyday life in the public service. The demands of the bureaucratic form of administration, the fragmented and specialised nature of many issues, the constraints on time, the limitations of resources and the secrecy surrounding new policy development all weigh heavily against consultation. Ministers may take the view that consultation with interest groups would be obstructive to their reform agenda, particularly when services are being reduced. However, it is clear that in many areas of public administration the development of program management has facilitated consultation between the public service and consumer groups by defining concrete topics for discussion centring around programs that have been proposed or are in progress.

The following sections consider some of the theoretical and practical issues involved in managing consumer consultation to enhance the instrumental operation of the public service. The issues are considered within the climate of Commonwealth government support for consultation, the strength of Australia's consumer organisations and peak councils, and the outcome-oriented program management of the Australian public service, none of which can be taken for granted. I conclude by arguing that consultation also has reflexive benefits for the ethos and policy skills within the public service itself.

MANAGING CONSUMER CONSULTATION

In attempting to formulate courses of action that may contribute to the public good, public administrators have always consulted with the public they serve. Of course, the particular forms and extent of these consultations have been determined by the modes of administration and the social structures of the day.

Reviews of consumer consultation undertaken before the widespread introduction of an overt managerialism with the public service in the 1980s emphasised the structure, roles and functions of the various consultative and advisory bodies set up by government, with particular concern for whether the representation on the bodies was fair and the procedures satisfactory. The Coombs Commission reviewed the structure and membership of all Commonwealth government advisory bodies, and analysed the interest group representation on these bodies (Coombs 1976, Appendixes 1L and 2D). Bailey assessed the workings of consultation through a review of 300 consultative arrangements between Commonwealth welfare departments and outside bodies (see Bailey et al. 1978, p. 208, for a summary list). These reviews played an important part in the scrutiny of public administration in the 1970s that formed the background for reform in the 1980s. It would be worthwhile repeating these empirical studies in the light of reforms since then.

However, with the widespread adoption of managerialism, the ground is shifting under the feet of such consultative bodies for two reasons. First, their importance has been overtaken by the growing strength and sophistication of non-government organisations representing both industry and consumers, and this has been encouraged by the Commonwealth government. These organisations, although frequently represented on government-constituted advisory bodies, have no compunction in pursuing their concerns through other channels such as the parliament, the media and the bureaucracy, including departments other than the one responsible for the advisory body. Second, many areas of the bureaucracy now develop specially tailored consultation strategies for individual policy initiatives and program components. These strategies frequently marginalise the influence of previously constituted advisory bodies.

While the advent of managerialism has sought to focus attention on outcomes, this is achieved by the creative and strategic use of the processes available to the public administration for particular policy initiatives or program components. Consumer consultation can be incorporated into a wide range of decision-making processes, from those involving the parliament and its committees, the cabinet and the budget cycle through to event planning and the delivery of services to end-users. In essence, good management of consumer consultation seeks to inject the insight and realism of consumer advocates into the processes of policy formation and program implementation.

Consultation can, of course, be disruptive to policy development and program implementation. In particular, there is the risk that the manager will lose control of the process. Much of the skill in managing consultation is in not allowing the consultation to derail the policy process or the program. Terry Slater, then a senior executive in the Commonwealth Department of Health, put this succinctly:

You have got to be careful not to throw away the management responsibility and management flexibility, not to give someone the right of veto over the content or the direction of how it is being managed, unless you deliberately want to do that. In framing the involvement of interested parties outside of the direct responsibility for implementation, one has to have it very clearly in mind what involvement you want from them (Dugdale 1992a, p. 277).

One judgment that needs to be made concerns the amount of time that can be assigned to consultation, and the extent of resources that need to be allocated for this to strike a balance between good consultation and effective policy development. To quote my colleague again:

You still [need] enough flexibility to meet the different situations that you are trying to consult or to deal with in an advocacy sense. I have felt the trade-off between time and cost in managing that process. Which means you want a policy out at a particular time, say to go into the budget process, and I've felt that the consultation process is another step in the critical path to achieve that work deadline and that work outcome. It is a trade-off in terms of whether to go ahead with a more elaborate or less elaborate or no consultation process (Dugdale 1992a, p. 282).

The question of who the consumers are and how they can be consulted is a vexed one, particularly at higher levels of government dealing with large-scale programs. It needs to be thought through in relation to each planned consultation, and there are no formulaic answers. The peak councils or their state counterparts are available as a starting place for discussion of this question. These include long-established organisations such as the Australian Council of Social Services (ACOSS) and the Australian Federation of Consumer Organisations (AFCO), more recently established groups such as the Consumers' Health Forum (CHF) and special-interest groups such as the Australian Federation of AIDS Organisations (AFAO), the Federation of Ethnic Community Councils of Australia (FECCA) and the Australian Council on the Ageing (ACOTA). The Australian Council of Trade Unions (ACTU) and the Business Council of Australia (BCA) can also be considered appropriate for this purpose. These groups can provide skilled advocates, can arrange contact with their member organisations, and can organise more direct 'grass-roots' consultations as appropriate. They can be an effective channel for accessing disadvantaged or stigmatised groups.

There are two debates concerning working with consumer organis-ations that should be mentioned. The first is the distinction between consumer and provider organisations. In some groups—for example, ACOSS—the distinction is not made, but in other groups the distinction is a point of principle, sometimes signified by including the word 'consumer' in their title (e.g. the Australian Federation of Consumer Organisations and the Consumers' Health Forum). The underlying sentiment of this debate is that the interests of providers and consumers are different, may conflict, and should not be confused. Although this difference can be overstated, sensitivities about the difference should be taken into account when deciding who to consult for a particular program.

The second debate is over whether a group receiving government fund-ing can be considered truly autonomous. On the one hand, acceptance of government funding always carries with it the threat of the funding being cut, and there is the possibility that groups may distract themselves by picking up funding for projects to which they are not primarily committed. On the other hand, business councils do not seem to worry about their reliance on the tax exemption that funds a considerable part of their contributions from members. In any case, it can be argued that the principal qualities to be looked for in consultations are insight and commitment to the sector of the community of concern to the program, not administrative autonomy.

In addition to program-planning exercises, consumer advocates can be used in program administration—for example, on advisory groups for grants programs, or on task-centred working groups. Some parts of the administration have a standing ministerial directive to include consumer representations on relevant intra-departmental committees and working groups, although of course what is relevant is the subject of continuing debate. The inclusion of consumer advocates on inter-departmental or inter-governmental committees can bring a dose of reality to the deliberations, and there may be advantages in suggesting this during the negotiations to set up these committees.

Perhaps the most common use of consumer consultation is in the evaluation of programs. This often takes the form of user surveys, and although these can be useful, more interactive forms of evaluation are a more creative source of ideas for improvement. Tensions may, however, arise between the rigid adherence to program objectives that will result in tighter evaluation, and flexibility of program objectives in response to consumer consultation. This tension is highlighted in evaluations that focus solely on the strategies used to achieve objectives and ignore evaluation of the objectives themselves.

Within any consultation itself, the advocates' hands cannot be tied and outcomes cannot be predicted. The manager needs to recognise that the concerns of the disadvantaged groups to which their programs are often directed are not intuitively apparent to public servants, no matter how public spirited they may be. The loss of control and increase in uncertainty on the part of the manager associated with consultation should be more than offset by the increased desirability of program outcomes and support for program strategies. Management satisfaction in the public sector should come not from the extent of control and influence wielded, but from the quality of the results achieved for the public benefit.

Engagement in consumer consultation is based on a view of the public service agency as open to influence by the public it serves. This requires a degree of control over actions and a concern with outcomes that can be enhanced considerably by program management techniques, an attitude of openness and accessibility of decision-making processes.

Managing consumer consultation also requires careful thought about structuring the channels of influence, including formal consultation and informal contact. Compared with consulting with other public sector agencies, consultation with consumers does not take place within common authority structures. In contrast to private sector consumer consultation, public sector consultation is framed by citizens' expectations of the public sector to act in their interests. The political nature of these consultations must be acknowledged openly.

Consumer consultation is fundamentally different from inter-departmental or inter-governmental consultation. Consulting with consumer groups is outside of the power and authority structures of the public administration and the parliament. There is not the shared under-standing that, at the end of the day, there are defined roles and responsibilities which frame the discussion and its outcomes.

In any inter-departmental negotiations, or with intra-departmental program negotiations, there is very much an organisational structure and a power structure—which at the end of the day, whether it is invoked or not, is always there.

With consumer groups or lobbyists, there isn't that understanding of where the group fits in and where they are coming from. So in this sense, discussions with advocates and outside bodies are not vastly different from discussions with private sector commercial firms. One has to under-stand what each party is seeking. Time must be taken to set out the expectations and agenda of both sides, and this may not be straightforward if either side lacks experience or if complex political issues are involved. Beforehand, it is important to understand what the group's agenda is and work out how that agenda might fit into the objectives of the program being sought, and of course with the government of the day's desires. And the government of the day's desires may well be to have that group satisfied. So in fact the consultations may well be about determining the agenda of that consumer group.

Clear understandings of the scope of the consultations need to be established at the outset. To avoid unrealistic expectations, the manager can project a picture of their own position in the bureaucracy with acknowledgment of their areas of responsibility and autonomy, but a con-servative estimate of their influence in other areas. It helps if all participants understand that, in general, the kinds of things that consumer groups want changed are difficult for the public administration to address, often requiring intersectoral action and high levels of public participation to be achieved.

As a rule, the closer to the grass-roots providers and consumers, the less the formal negotiating skills. The manager's role in consultations is that of a facilitator, providing information and structure where appropriate without railroading the discussions to a predetermined conclusion. In a sense, through consultation the manager becomes a participant in community discussions, and these in turn can be brought into close relation to bureaucratic policy development and the machinations of government.

The development of the National Women's Health Policy in the late 1980s (Commonwealth DCSH 1989a) illustrates some of the dynamics of this process. The Women's Health Network had a large input to a report which very much reflected its agenda but which the responsible manager in the Commonwealth Department of Health judged would have been difficult for the government of the day to consider because it didn't have the polish, the breadth of view of the issues, or the wherewithal to get government support—particularly in terms of funding. There was considerable delicacy in ensuring that ownership was retained while shaping the document to produce the outcomes the government wanted in a way which would win cabinet support.

The manager put in place, over and above the women's sub-committee that the Australian Health Ministers Advisory Council had set up, a departmental steering committee which he chaired and which had on it the chairperson of the women's sub-committee. She was quite crucial, and her credibility, of course, was on the line—within the women's network, not within the department.

With each succeeding draft the departmental committee went through, any changes went back to be debated by the sub-committee of AHMAC so that it could see the changes. Towards the end, with the minister focusing on it, a very sharp thrust for that policy came out—about establishing community women's health centres—which in the original document hadn't assumed an importance or focus. The departmental committee then had to come back and refocus the document. Because of the goodwill and the trust and the understanding that had been built up, it went through with a minimum of fuss.

This example illustrates the delicacy required for interpolating the realism of community advocates into hard-edged new policy development. Ultimately, the policy and budget arena of the Commonwealth government operates with highly stylised texts and bizarre patterns of negotiation. Admitting the lay public to the processes involved requires a large amount of effort on the part of the bureaucracy. It presents an enormous technical challenge to management, and is outside their experience with the processes of intra-governmental consultation.

Public sector consultation with consumer groups is also fundamentally different from consultation between private sector agencies and consumers. In the private sector, the pursuit of profit provides a clear reference point and the main competition is between providers. In the public sector, there is no universal reference point and the main competition is between consumers, who often have expectations of the public sector based on traditions of public service and the rights of citizens. Put another way, public sector consultation with community groups should be about empowerment and reducing the disadvantages of those consulted with, not about making a profit from them.

Because the provision of public services is part of governmental politics, and because of the interrelations of party political agendas and consumer advocate agendas, public sector consultation with consumers is an inherently political activity. It involves careful balancing of competing groups and divergent interests, and a search for consensus based on the development of trust and understanding, creative discussion of possible courses of action, and a willingness to compromise. To effectively manage those dynamics and processes, managers must openly acknowledge the political nature of the consultation. This includes addressing the role of politicians in the discussions. For example, is the minister to be involved by agreeing to the consultation plan, or by personally attending a consultation meeting? Are other politicians to be involved, including opposition spokespersons and members of parliamentary committees?

The politics of the consumer groups themselves are perhaps less weighty than those of the parliamentary arena, but they are complex nevertheless, and marked by a shifting and amorphous character. Consumer advocates are rarely elected by consumers, but can usually mobilise considerable support for their positions if pressed. This is particularly true of office holders and employees of the national peak councils, who generally have well-developed links with the media. The manager involved in consultation should seek to understand the background of the consumer advocates and their relationship to the target group, just as they must understand their own place in the bureaucracy. The interests of the advocate need to be taken into account, and these personal interests are quite different from the interests on whose behalf they are advocating. There is a fine line between what is ideologically acceptable in a consensus sense to the group, and what could be important to leading members of the group—there is a difference because of other agendas. Leading members may well be those who need to be targeted first, and got on side. Advocates may be elected office holders of small organisations, respected ideologues, committed time servers or charismatic community figures. An understanding of where advocates are coming from will help the manager interpret their position in discussions.

If possible, consultation discussions should be kept concrete. In policy and planning discussions, a focus on target groups and client needs often performs this function. It must be kept in mind, however, that the community rarely organises itself neatly around the ascriptive criteria used to define target groups. For example, if a program is to be directed at people with asthma, then asthma self-help groups cannot be ignored. However, it should be recognised that each person with asthma spends most of their time in their household, workplace or place of education, and that their main support comes from their family and friends, not other people with asthma. This has been recognised by many in the self-help movement, and underlies the preference for active signifiers such as 'people with asthma' or 'people living with AIDS' over passive forms such as 'asthmatics' or 'AIDS victims'.

Problems of over-intervention are particularly hard to identify and can be politically unpalatable to address, but there is no doubt that, as in the private sector, competition between public sector agencies is occurring for the privilege of providing services to clients. Consultation can highlight the wide-ranging interactions of programs with other services—state and federal, public and private. In consultation about existing services or programs, a focus on the perceived problems of the service can identify overlaps and facilitate planning for remedial action. I have mentioned the possibility of conflict between providers and consumers of services. More frequently, providers and consumers develop a codependency that can interfere with the critical evaluation of services. This often-unconscious collusion can include tolerance of lax cost controls, inadequate targeting of resources and provider acquiescence to client demands outside the intention of the program.

Consultation is based on a commitment to dialogue that can take the concerns of consumers to the heart of program administration. The establishment of this dialogue requires trust, built up in a wider framework than the specific consultation itself. As in any interaction, cooperation with a consumer group is a two-way street. The manager needs to consider this cooperation in a wider framework than the immediate consultation.

Consultation with a consumer group can itself promote community development as an intended or unintended (but desirable!) side-effect. Support for consumer advocacy groups can include:

- providing funding to cover the cost of consultation;
- providing funding for infrastructure. Consumer organisational costs are relatively low, but the cost of accountability needs to be built in;
- supporting organisational and personnel development. Strategies can include conference attendance, staff exchange and use of organisational consultants, although these latter strategies may engender controversy;
- funding research. This should take into account the research agenda of both the funding body and the recipient;
- providing information on policy activities with the opportunity for informal input.

Successful consultation requires accessibility and commitment to feedback. One problem that may be encountered is that, for a variety of reasons, including the time taken for decisions made through consultation to have an impact, consumer advocates are not good at communicating the result of consultations back to their constituencies. Peak councils are expert at translating the experiences of their constituents into generalised terms for policy debates, but are much less able to explain what policy decisions mean to the constituents. People relay their experience, they don't generalise to what that actually means in a policy form. There is a circle that goes on where the peak councils actually have to generalise that up so it has meaning in terms of national policy and national legislation. They then should go back through that grass-roots constituency to explain what policy positions mean what, in terms of what people want. They don't do that very well.

A final point to make is that there are dangers if the decision to consult with consumer organisations is taken lightly. Consultation distracts from the core activities of the group and members may be disillusioned, with there being little to show for previous consultative efforts. It is counterproductive to engage in a mechanical consultative process so that government can say its policies have been developed in consultation and the full-time lobbyists can report to their clients that their voice was heard by government.

I would like to conclude by discussing an old but useful debate concerning the nature and importance of policy in public sector management. The concern has arisen as the generic manager has been privileged over the subject expert in senior public service management. John Uhr (1987), among others, has noted the decline of emphasis on policy skills in public service management training, giving rise to the fear that this aspect of public service may become ineffective: 'our quest for efficiencies of resource management might well lead to disturbing new levels of ineffectiveness in a vital end product of public policy—advice and evaluation of public policy' (1987, p. 375).

Peter Wilenski (1988), a Commonwealth departmental head (and, interestingly, a medical practitioner), did not believe that this was a cause for concern, but did outline his own concern about the interrelation between the instrumental operation of the public service and the implementation of public service values. He points out that, in contrast to the instrumental view of the public service as 'a neutral machine that mechanically put policy into effect' (Wilenski 1988, p. 217), managers must go beyond the dichotomy of policy-making and policy implementation. Failure to take this view could leave the managerialist with an approach that is too instrumental and with the problem of insensitivity to the community. Progressive public administrators have:

> discarded the policy–administration dichotomy and begun to realise that each act of administration defines and refines 'policy' and is itself 'policy-making' activity. It requires the exercise of value judgements . . . The new managerialism for all its virtues may become unduly mechanistic and, like the old instrumentalism, may have an unconscious bias which will make it difficult for disadvantaged groups to deal with the bureaucracy, to obtain their fair share of programs (1988, pp. 217–18).

I have argued throughout this discussion that consumer consultation contributes to better policy and better administration in the interrelated sense of the terms spelt out by Wilenski, and that it provides a route of access for citizens—including disadvantaged groups—to influence the bureaucracy and the management of public sector programs. However, this does not happen automatically. Management of consultation for maximum effectiveness requires a high level of traditional policy skills, including conceptual clarity in presenting the issues for consultation and in documenting the understandings reached; accurate analysis of the consequences of programs and proposals under discussion; appreciation of linkages between items under discussion and their wider social context; political insight; and a feel for the wider policy agenda.

The techniques of managerialism can, of course, be extremely helpful in this—for example, in using sophisticated accounting systems to calculate resource implications, or using program statements of objectives and strategies as a framework for documenting understandings reached on what needs changing. Ensuring there is good representation of people with a high level of policy skills in consultations can help avoid problems such as continually going over old ground, going off on unproductive tangents or the discontinuities that may be caused by turnover of participants. Many consumer advocates will themselves have considerable policy skills, and these can be utilised to good effect in consultations where a cooperative ethos has been established.

Consumer consultation is a particular area of activity for the public sector, with its own set of considerations, techniques, pitfalls and rewards. To be successful, it requires senior management involvement if only because of its political character. I have tried to show that consumer consultation stands to benefit from a variety of managerialist innovations. More importantly, it makes an important contribution to good public management. By highlighting equity issues and policy skills, a commitment to consumer consultation guards against some of the more serious potential problems raised by the managerialist tendencies inherent in our modern large bureaucracies.

POLICY ACTIVISM

The remainder of this chapter explores policy activism by people working in government agencies. It discusses policy activism in the field of health to show how the governmentality of the health system relates to the social activism and lived experience of people working for change within the health system.

I begin with a definitional discussion and consider who might be the policy activists working inside the health system. I then examine the ethics of policy activism inside government: I draw a distinction between transcendent and immanent activism, and argue that the latter is more helpful for understanding the activism of the insider. This is illustrated by considering the ethics of the public health professional working inside a government agency, and asking how they may operate as an insider policy activist. Out of the constraints, privileges, powers and concerns associated with activists in different institutional and community locations, a division of activist labour emerges: insider activists become oriented to different deployments of their activism than community-based activists. There are two activist technologies, or 'power tools', that can be wielded by insider activists in the analysis of the policy discourse. These focus on the governmentality of the health system by showing what there is to be done and how to do it, and in this way open up opportunities to use policy to produce social change. Insider activists are concerned with the historical permutations of policy debates for the identification of activist goals, and the possibilities that arise in the enunciation of policy statements for the pursuit of those goals. These matters are illustrated below by considering some of the major features of Australia's health system in the Medicare era.

The chapter concludes with an examination of the relationship between insider activists and the institutions within which they work, and reflects on the impact of the institutional environment on the subjective experience of insider activism. As I wrote each description of activism in this chapter, I held in mind a particular person I considered to be a policy activist inside the health system. I have not sought their corroboration of the analyses I ascribe to their situations. They are by nature, and force of circumstance, shy about their activism, so it would be wrong of me to identify them; however, in most cases acknowledgment of their contributions has come from elsewhere.

There is a distinction between policy activists based in the community and policy activists based inside government agencies. Both words in the term 'policy activist' present problems in their definition. However, for community-based activists the major difficulty lies in locating their participation in the policy process, whereas for the insider activist the difficulty lies in deciding whether they are an activist or not. We can readily accept that outsiders who do participate in the policy process are activists, for who but an activist would engage in policy work? Inside government, for people routinely working in and around policy processes, the main difficulty is to work out what we mean by 'activist'. If they are an activist, they can readily be defined as policy activists. But what would make them an activist?

The German sociologist Max Weber (1978) offers some clues in his consideration of politics as a vocation written in 1919. In this essay, he considers what type of person would find politics a viable vocation. Weber identifies the following characteristics: an urge for power, an attitude of detachment to facilitate good judgment, and a passion for a realistic cause. The characteristics that suit a person for the vocation of public service are on the surface markedly different: an eye for detail, respect for authority, a sense of fairness. Nevertheless, the bureaucracy may attract the activist, and may nurture activism amongst those working within it. Weber himself spent more time analysing the bureaucracy than the polity, and actually spent a year or so as administrator of Germany's military hospital system (Runciman 1978, p. xii). Much of what he discusses in 'Politics as a vocation' is applicable to a career in public service with an activist orientation. In this chapter, I have adapted two of Weber's themes, specifically his concern with the ethics of deploying state power for the good of the people, and an insistence that the capacity to sustain a reasonable cause is central to activism as a vocation (Weber 1978, pp. 216–18).

As an undergraduate, I was involved in student politics. During a reflective discussion on what the future would hold—taking place in the campus tavern—an activist colleague declared that when he left the political nursery of the university he wanted to become a faceless bureaucrat with multi-million dollar budgets to play with. The attraction was the realistic chance of achieving something worthwhile. He had no hankering after fame or recognition, having had a small taste of it on campus. Looking to the bureaucracy, he saw the hierarchical organisation and the cross-linking to the policies of the elected government as potential means to be worked with for activist ends—a counter-intuitive perception for most young outsider activists. My friend did indeed become a career bureaucrat with a policy orientation. Over the last two decades, as an insider activist, he has been intimately involved in the struggle to produce progressive health, social and market policy in both Commonwealth and state departments, under both Labor and Liberal/National Coalition governments.

Alternatively, rather than bringing their activism with them, people may develop an activist orientation through working in government agencies. Health professionals working in service delivery may take up the cause of their client group, and try to influence policy on their behalf (social workers have even defined such advocacy as one of their professional competencies). People working in health policy may develop a commitment to particular issues on which they are working. Public health professionals providing technical input to policy development may become passionate about the policy outcome and broaden their engagement in the policy process well beyond the role of expert. For these transformations to count as orientations to activism, the primary motivation must be compassionately directed towards the people the policy governs, not towards furthering the career of the insider.

It may be more or less easy to be an insider activist at different times and in different agencies. Activists may follow a trajectory that moves in and out of the bureaucracy, and this is facilitated by a professional or academic background. While one's activism may often be at odds with the policy orientation and operational style of a particular agency, there are many occasions where there is considerable affinity between the two. For example, the government of the day may adopt attitudes to policy matters advocated by community-based activists, and then ask for these to be progressed by specific government agencies. Community-based activists may be appointed to senior positions within the agency because of government support for their stance. Learning to be an effective operator in the bureaucratic jungle then becomes a particular cross to bear for these outsiders-turned-insiders.

Insiders with an orientation to policy activism may demonstrate their activism by working in many ways. They may build networks of relationships across government agencies and with outsiders who share their cause or activist leanings. They may go beyond the brief of their allocated work and push for their cause. They may weight their time towards progressing their activist interests at the expense of other work. They may argue their cause passionately with their superiors against the latter's expressed preferences. All of these ways of working carry a risk to the insider that they are prepared to take on due to their activist commitments. This brings us to a discussion of the practical ethics of insider activism.

The characteristics of insider activism have much in common with the way health professionals in general conduct themselves within government agencies. The latter's profession provides a platform for the formation of policy priorities external to government. The process of becoming a professional also confers a sense of primary allegiance by the professional to the profession that is not easily supplanted. There are also accepted styles of personal conduct developed by professionals, including a capacity and willingness to stand up for one's professional autonomy. Nevertheless, despite some shared characteristics, professionalism (as a health professional) within government agencies is different from activism, particularly concerning the activist professional's motivations and relationship to the community.

It is unlikely that one could formulate an essential definition of the activist or activism. However, activism can be characterised along a number of dimensions. First, activism specifies action, and the distribution of social arenas within which this action takes place can be used to characterise various types of activism: political activism, specifying action within political arenas; welfare activism, specifying action within the welfare sector; or policy activism, specifying action in the policy process. Second, activism implies a cause, and the distribution of causes can be used to characterise various types of activism: human rights activism is concerned with human rights; environmental activism is concerned with the environment. Third, various types of people are activists, and the distribution of ascriptive groups can be used to characterise various types of activists: black activists, feminist activists, disabled activists or HIV-positive activists.

The final dimension of activism is one I shall consider in more detail. It concerns the origin of the activist's motivation. The cause of the activism can arise immanently from within the field of action itself, or transcendentally from some other sphere. The archetype of the transcendent activist would be the Christian missionaries trying to bring about the Kingdom of God on earth. These are people who receive their mission as a vocation from an authority that has no relation to the place or situation where they are going to go and be activists. They then take that mission to the local people. Once *in situ*, they may well look for local causes to pursue compassionately with the local people for the greater glory of God. Other examples could include the revolutionary Marxist or some single-issue social movement activists. The key feature of transcendent activists is that they receive their view of what is to be done quite independently from the field where it is to be done.

For immanent activists, there is no transcendental rupture between their motivation and their actions. Both find their cause in the situation at hand, however broadly that is perceived. From an immanent perspective, you cannot know what it is possible to do until you are in a position to do it. It is only by immersing yourself in the circumstances of the field with which you are concerned that you can recognise the possibilities for action and achievement available from the position in which you find yourself.

Consider two examples of the immanent activist. First, there is the female medical practitioner who stands for election to her AMA branch council and gets elected on a vote relating to the need for new blood; however, once in position she has to actually determine what is to be done. She will no doubt be aware of the cultural tensions within the profession as it drags its feet towards the future, but she cannot know until actually elected what the possibilities that would allow her to make a difference might be. Second, what of the bureaucrat in the public service who, after a restructure, finds himself in a new branch that didn't exist previously? Initially, he may not even know what the branch's role is. But with a commitment to doing something progressive, he sets about working out the possibilities of what can be done from an activist perspective, as the work program of the branch develops.

Transcendentally motivated activism has a long and distinguished history. However, I would contend that the contemporary environment of government agencies in the health system—or indeed the public sector more broadly—lends itself more readily to engagement by an immanent activism. In support of this contention, let me offer a more sustained illustration of the immanent ethics of insider policy activism by considering the public health professional working in the public health system. Public health, replete with its multidisciplinary diversity, has always been central to health policy formation. The influence of public health doctors on the development of government Departments of Health from 1910 to 1960 has been documented by James Gillespie in his book *The Price of Health* (1991). During the 1970s, the influence of public health professionals on the action of government health agencies declined. This was partly due to a diminishing perception of the importance of traditional core activities of public health such as communicable disease surveillance and control, partly due to a purge of medically qualified people from management positions in Commonwealth and state health departments, and partly because of the lack of an external professional base for public health professionals outside government agencies at this time.

During the 1980s, public health experienced a considerable renaissance, relating to the 'new public health' movement that developed under the auspices of the World Health Organization (WHO 1986), the expansion of the Public Health Association, the creation of the Faculty of Public Health Medicine within the Royal Australasian College of Physicians, the development of popular Masters of Public Health courses in many universities, and the expansion of public health and related units within the major health bureaucracies. The improved professional organisation of public health and the growth in numbers of public health professionals within government agencies has greatly expanded the conditions of possibility for an engagement by these people in the policy process. Let us now tease out how this can occur, and examine the differences and overlaps between professional conduct and activism in the policy process.

Involvement of public health professionals in the policy process is often based on deploying their technical skills and expert knowledge within the process. Technical skills include facility with statistical methods, information technology, field surveillance, and disease prevention or control. Expert knowledge includes historical and contemporary patterns of disease development and medical response at the population level. These skills and knowledges are based on a strong interdisciplinary academic structure encompassing biostatistics, demography and epidemiology, together with the more recent emergence of health promotion, public administration and health economics interests within public health.

At the more general level, public health professionals have an interest in policy because of the potential for the policy process to bring about a greater level of health or well-being in the community. Because of their skills and knowledge, public health professionals are valuable within policy processes. But at whose instigation, and what type of contribution can they make? Public health professionals are often brought into the policy process solely for their skills. Many of us have had the experience of being used in a piecemeal fashion, being asked to extract statistics on this or that topic, with no clear idea of how the information will be used. Perhaps this is acceptable for the disinterested policy professional.

Activist professionals strive to actively join in policy processes as they arise, and may seek to stimulate debate and policy development in line with their activist motivations. They can be distinguished by the active deployment of their usefulness to gain access to the key decision-making forums within policy processes of interest to them as activists, with the aim of realising some substantive goals. In the pursuit of influence on the policy process, the activist professional is faced with the task of determining the relevance of public health knowledges and techniques to the debate at hand, with a view to maximising his or her own involvement and that of sympathetic professional colleagues. Closely related to this, the activist professional needs to develop an understanding of the various agencies, relationships and perspectives involved, and reflect on whether it would be helpful to involve other agencies or seek representation from those who will be receiving the services under discussion.

Such a pragmatic approach marks the activist professional as different from the usual image of the professional within the policy process. Professionals are often considered by senior bureaucrats (with good grounds) to be captured by their own profession's interests, unwilling to venture beyond the bounds of their professional expertise and uninterested in the concerns and perspectives of other policy actors, particularly non-professional ones. The professional and activist orientations converge in a synergistic way when the activist professional pursues a rational, empirically informed approach, takes the trouble to understand diverging interests in the policy process, and attempts to keep the focus on the optimum structure, coordination and operation of the health system in its efforts to improve the health of the public.

I have suggested that a defining characteristic of the policy activist health professional working inside a government agency is that they act on causes arising from outside the agency, and concerned with some aspect of the health system itself. These causes may be restricted to a single issue, such as the provision of services to people with HIV/AIDS, or increasing support for relatives who care for the chronically ill. In my experience, however, single-issue insider activists are rare: most are quite broadly committed to pursuing progressive change in the health system. This broader, immanent orientation develops over time for any insider who maintains an activist orientation, even if it first emerged as a transcendent single-issue concern.

So what do insider policy activists actually do? I propose that a division of activist labour has emerged between community-based policy activists and insider policy activists. A preliminary specification of the components of policy activist work might include: identification of causes for activists in a form that can be taken up in the policy discourse; the raising of issues on governmental policy agendas; provoking community debate on issues; involving political parties in the cause; determining policy processes through which the cause can be pursued; and using the policy process to deliver on the cause. The components of this list can be formulated in many different ways, and may vary from issue to issue and sector to sector.

My main purpose in describing a division of activist labour is not to pigeonhole either activists or their activities, but to facilitate a discussion of how various aspects of activist work relate to various parts of the policy process. However, it must be kept in mind that there can be many exceptions, and some activists for whom it is difficult to say whether they are located in the community or in a government agency. There are constraints on the activities of employees of government agencies that have implications for which aspects of policy activism they can pursue. They should not publicly undermine the government of the day. They should not criticise existing government policies in the field in which they work, except as part of government-instigated reviews of those policies. They should not provide opposition parties with the means of political advantage, except through formal government channels using official processes of communication.

These constraints apply to government employees, whether working directly with policy or not. They generally apply only within the person's direct field of work. People who ignore these constraints risk being formally disciplined (including being demoted or sacked) or informally kept away from policy processes. There are ways around the constraints, to do with the rights of government employees to participate as citizens in the processes of government. For example, unions or professional associations may provide protected forums in which to speak out and engage in public activities. Political parties may provide closed and protected forums for airing discontent. However, these ways around the constraints imposed in working for government agencies are generally not useful for people in management positions or those working explicitly in the policy process. These constraints are constraints on insider activism. There are other constraints on activism by people within non-government organisations who receive government funding, or individuals and organisations who wish to enter into and maintain a formal dialogue with government (see Papadakis 1984, pp. 204–8; Dugdale 1992a, pp. 99–106).

Such constraints determine the differences and the division of labour between insider policy activists and community-based activists. For example, community-based activists must take the running on provoking community debate (e.g. by staging public demonstrations) and fuelling political point scoring by opposition parties. These activities are things the insider activist usually avoids. The two things that insider policy activists can do, that are virtually impossible for people who do not think in terms of the governmentality of the health system, who have not had hands-on policy experience, are to locate issues in contemporary policy debates and to map a path through the policy process. These are what we might call the activist technologies or 'power tools' of policy activism available to the insider activist, based on the personal know-how, the knowledge and culture of the deep throat policy analyst.

The ability to analyse contemporary debates can be useful for enabling the activist network to strategically tune itself for maximum relevance and effectiveness. The knowledge of how to chart a course through the policy process can help convert activist energies into social change. These two sets of know-how make the insider policy activist highly sought after by both community-based and political activists, and confer a certain mystique on the insider (compounded, no doubt, by the somewhat monastic work habits their institutional environments demand). The next two sections consider these activist technologies in more detail.

READING POLICY DEBATE

Specific health policy issues which can form the ground for insider activism arise in the health policy discourse from the material, historical features of the health system. The first activist technology I consider concerns how to bring these issues to light in such a way that they can be addressed through the policy process. This section considers the possibilities for insider policy activism in the Medicare era in relation to some of the major features in the terrain of health policy since the introduction of Medicare. The case study aims to show how to 'use political practice as an intensifier of thought and analysis as a multiplier of the forms and domains for the intervention of political action' (Foucault 1983).

In 1983–84, the newly elected Hawke Labor government brought in the Medicare policy. As previously discussed, the Medicare policy centred around global funding for the health system to be provided by the Commonwealth in order to drive clear objectives for the health system, in particular to provide a comprehensive health system for everybody in Australia. Ever since, numerous difficulties and caveats have intervened in the translation of that simple policy approach to the complex reality of the contemporary health system.

The introduction of a major new policy initiative, such as the creation of a new national health system, extinguishes one series of debates and creates the possibility of a whole new set. The debates that used to be had in health policy, before the introduction of Medicare, were quite different from contemporary debates and have effectively run their course or been profoundly transformed. Consider two examples. First, debates on whether a new hospital should be built in a particular area used to turn mainly on political considerations ('porkbarrelling') because there was no real capacity to enunciate the equitable geographical distribution of health facilities as a clear objective. Second, the debate concerning the functional importance of private health insurance and how to increase coverage rates has been transformed by everybody in Australia getting public health insurance coverage, because this fundamentally changed the nature of private health insurance as a product, turning it from a basic necessity needed to avoid financial ruin into a luxury product.

The new debates which have emerged since the early 1980s include at least three main themes: the boundaries of the Medicare system; equity issues; and the adequacy of the health system. Each theme has been associated with a whole series of activist causes.

The first set of debates concerns what are to be the boundaries within which the health system provides services for the population. Does the health system include aged care? Should comprehensive health care include looking after people's teeth, providing podiatrist services for foot care, or providing financial support for carers? Should Medicare benefits be available for allied health services such as psychology and physiotherapy? Should psychiatric services be kept separate or mainstreamed into the acute medical care system (NSW Health Department 1993)? These boundary issues have been hard fought over the last two decades. In many cases, intelligence from insider policy activists has been crucial to the efficient coordination of efforts within activist networks in identifying and supporting particular causes.

The introduction of Medicare also created the possibility for a new set of debates on equity in relation to reform of the health system. From the early 1970s until 1984, the central debate in the party political arena had been concerned with the differential access to health services experienced by people of varying socioeconomic status (e.g. see Opit 1984). Following the introduction of Medicare, the concern for equality of access permutated into a concern with the differential access to health facilities by people from different geographical areas. This concern for geographical equity has since become a driver of change in the state hospital systems (Macklin 1991).

Gough Whitlam had foreshadowed this in the early 1970s when, according to health policy folklore, he made a pronouncement from the roof of the MLC Tower (then the highest building in Sydney) along the following lines: looking below us, we see a community served by one of the greatest collections of hospitals in the industrialised world; looking to western Sydney, we see two million people living with one of the poorest. The development of Liverpool, Westmead and Nepean hospitals since then has transformed this.

From a policy perspective, the introduction of the Medicare national health system in 1983/84 (following the halting progress and demise of Medibank from 1975—see Scotton and MacDonald 1993; Wooldridge 1991) provided the political impetus for a concrete focus on equity of access to health services. Needs-based planning had already achieved the status of the dominant approach to hospital and health service development by the early 1980s (see Sax 1984). During the 1980s, with the introduction of a new managerialism into the Australian Public Service (for a review of this, see Considine and Painter 1997), this evolved into a funding formula-based approach in most state health systems. By the mid-1990s, all states and territories had divided health services into geographical areas, and most now fund those areas on the basis of a formula that takes into account the population in the area and its health service needs.

From a health system perspective, the permutation in the expression of equality-based reform objectives from a concern with socioeconomic status to a concern with geographical location can partly be explained by the injection of increased cashflow into the public health system in the early years of Medicare. Combined with the increase in the number of people entitled to free care in the public hospital system, the recurrent cash injection led to a refocusing of concern about under-funding in the health system away from recurrent budgets and on to the need for increased capital to renovate, upgrade and expand the network of public hospitals. This opened up the tension between refurbishing existing hospitals versus building new ones in relatively under-resourced areas, a cause taken up by many health policy activists, particularly in Sydney. At the same time, the new managerialist approach to global funding of health services, in the context of universal health service coverage for the whole population, made possible the enunciation of equitable geographical access as a central objective for health system program development at the national level.

Medicare also introduced the possibility of a new set of debates about the adequacy of the health system. These have taken at least three specific forms. Is Medicare doing enough for enough people? Is the health system keeping up with new technology? Is Australia saddled with a system from 1983 that is unable to respond to events within health services, to developments within the health professions and to emerging diseases? Each of these debates has provided the ground for health policy activist claims to be formulated and pursued. Consider the following examples.

A community-based campaign took place in the second half of the 1980s around the inadequacy of the health system for disabled people, with Disabled Persons International being a notable focal point for community-based activists. There were a number of insider activists involved in Commonwealth and several state health departments. This activism found a policy expression in the development and implementation of the Commonwealth–State Disability Agreements (for a review, see Yeatman 1996), which were based around the partitioning of disability services from mainstream health services.

The HIV/AIDS pandemic, brought to light in the early 1980s, was the first major test of the responsiveness of the new Medicare health system to a dramatic new global health problem. It brought together a wide range of activists across the gay community, the medical profession, the universities, the Commonwealth Health Department, and the parliament. The Labor health minister who had rung in the Medicare system—and thus had an enormous amount riding on a demonstration of the new system's capacity to cope with an emerging epidemic of this magnitude—assumed leadership and encouraged the activists. The response was spectacularly successful, although paradoxically this was achieved by developing a disease-specific response nested within the general public insurance health system. This strategic move itself was no doubt partially responsible for fostering a sense of activism amongst the participants, close but strange bedfellows that they were to become.

Finally, one of the major adequacy debates created by the nationalisation of the health system concerns the size of the pie—the total amount of resources to be provided to the Australian public health system. This new policy object drew on and integrated various lower level debates on adequacy in health services as well as the issue of the equitable distribution of facilities. Whether the pie was big enough at the national level was a question that could not really be addressed until we had a national health system to answer for. Once this debate opened up, it almost immediately ramified into the discourse on fiscal policy and multiplied the strategies available for health policy activism. Activists could accept the challenge of debating fiscal policy, and argue the benefits to community welfare that flow from public sector health financing against the orthodox tendency within the fiscal discourse towards smaller government. Alternatively, they could accept 'fiscal constraints' and direct their activism towards cost-neutral reform options concerning the redistribution of resources. Many policy activists, of course, pursued both these strategies simultaneously (interestingly, insider activists were less likely to accept the strange argument that no growth was good growth in health financing because health expenditure growth was bad for the economy).

Within the framework of a national, globally funded public sector health system, these debates provide a wide range of opportunities for health policy activism that would not have made sense before the introduction of Medicare. Their emergence has created the conditions of possibility for health policy activism in the Medicare era for both community-based and insider activists. The discussion in this section has sought to bring out some of the opportunities for activism that arise in the health policy discourse and the role insider activists play in following this discourse and identifying such opportunities.

WRITING POLICY

I turn now to how policy insiders actually deliver results by considering the way the enunciation of policy brings about its effects. Knowing how to frame policy statements so they actually make a positive difference is the second power tool wielded by the insider policy activist. It is one of the most difficult and prized arts of government, and its application by the insider activist is both a highly political practice and a great intensifier of thought.

The development and deployment of administrative technologies for governing represent a rapidly changing field. Introduction of a new technique can bring in its wake a profound reorganisation of institutional structures, relationships, roles and responsibilities. Program budgeting and the purchaser–provider split are two well-known examples (Keating 1988; Boston 1995). A changed approach to governing, and the associated alterations to the institutional terrain they usher in, change the way activist causes can be articulated just as much as the introduction of a major new policy or program. The introduction of new technologies of government changes the way activist causes can be pursued.

Policy is an immanent or emergent reality arising out of the policy process, or more broadly the concrete government of a social field. The processes of idea formation, implementation and uptake are articulated as a policy discourse encompassing the politics, knowledges, action and relationships it assembles. In this context, specific policies are enunciated as statements of government. Enunciation of statements within the policy discourse is performed by a range of policy actors (not just 'the government'), each of whom occupies a number of subject positions (they talk of the different hats they wear) within a vast array of institutional locations. Policy statements are events that function to make sense of the broad policy field in particular ways. They are made over and over again throughout the policy process from development to implementation, in endlessly related permutations that determine the interpretation and actions of the policy in a proliferating array of sites. Policy statements can be analysed by considering the objects which the policy governs, the subject positions from which the policies are enunciated and the conceptual fields the policy statements occur within. These three domains then constitute the strategic terrain for the activities of people who work with policy, including insider policy activists.

Let us now examine how such an analysis can be developed by again considering the Resource Distribution Formula (RDF) of the New South Wales Health Department. During the 1980s, the operational units of the New South Wales health system—hospitals, community health centres, public health services and the like—were organised into geographically defined comprehensive health services. These have varied in number and changed their names over the years. At the time of writing, there are eight area health services covering New South Wales. Resources made available by the New South Wales government for various statewide health service programs (including population health services, primary and community-based services, acute inpatient services and mental health services) are allocated each year according to the RDF. As discussed in Chapter 4, the formula takes account of the number of people in the area; their health needs as calculated according to their age distribution and modified by factors for Aboriginality, homelessness and poor English speaking; and their utilisation of private health services. The area/district health services then distribute the resources they receive to health service provider agencies (such as hospitals and community health centres), both inside and outside their area, to provide services for the population residing within their area.

How is the RDF to be understood as a series of policy statements in terms of its object, subject, conceptual and strategic domains? First, the object of policy cannot be conceived as independent from the policy itself. It is not a matter of picking out some pre-existing set of social arrangements as an object to be governed. The object of the policy is actually constructed through the delineation of a social reality—a reality that may not have meaningful existence for policy until the policy has been constructed. Second, the subject position from which a policy is to be enunciated needs to be analysed and understood. Who is speaking, who is enunciating the policy, and what are the characteristics of the space they occupy as a subject? These are all questions that need to be asked by the health policy activist looking to try to make a difference.

The object directly governed by the RDF is the set of dollar amounts which are to be provided to the area health services. This set has a number of properties, enunciated in the New South Wales government's *Economic Statement for Health* (NSW Government 1995a), and subsequent policy statements and budget documents which frame the formula—principally that the dollar amounts will be calculated as a share of available funds, and that these amounts are for a population of people, not a collection of health facilities. The New South Wales Health Department—a different corporate entity from the government, responsible to but separate from the minister of health—has enunciated the actual set of dollar amounts by elaborating these principles into a statement of the detailed mathematical form which the formula is to take, and providing guidance on the operational implications it has for area/district health services. All of these statements contribute to the delineation of the object governed by the RDF, along with myriad unpublished letters, memos and the like produced by policy officers, area CEOs, finance officers and so on: a great field of opportunity for insider policy activists. Addressing fairness under the RDF regime is a question of the form of the RDF. The potential for activism derives from the responsiveness to the need for change that a mechanism like the RDF confers on the New South Wales public health system.

Third, policy statements are enunciated within a conceptual web of other governmental statements and debates that make up the health policy discourse. Concerning the RDF, this web includes the New South Wales and Commonwealth governments' fiscal policies; the prevailing way of doing business in the New South Wales public sector through a cascading series of performance contracts between minister and department, department and area health service, area health service and hospital, and hospital and clinical unit (for an analysis of this form of public sector contractualism, see Yeatman 1995); policies to deal with waiting lists which in the past have required a retreat from resource redistribution due to the short-term inefficiencies it produces; policies concerning people from non-English speaking backgrounds, and so on. Activist causes present in any of these fields can be pursued in relation to the RDF. It can readily be seen that the intersection of more or less related issues and policy mechanisms is often extremely complex. In particular, specific administrative technologies such as the RDF carry the implementation of many disparate sets of objectives, some of which may conflict. In this kind of situation, a role for the insider policy activist emerges around brokering the way different causes—activist, administrative, political—can be articulated with the governmental technology at hand.

Finally, on the matter of strategy, it is important to recognise the deep entwinedness of power and knowledge. Part of the struggle within policy work is to promote particular forms of expertise over others. The knowledge that forms the basis for a new policy field reflects the sedimentation of the power struggles that went into the construction of that field. The RDF is based on a social strategy. It represents the outcome of the struggle of policy activists championing the cause of social justice through equitable resource distribution. However, it also presents an opportunity for activists with other agendas to operate across the new governmental terrain opened up by the RDF with its associated structures and processes. For example, those aligned with public health may argue in the area health service annual budget policy cycle for a greater share of resources to go to health promotion.

A number of actors affect the construction and operation of funding formulas. These include the people who are enumerated in the calculation of population number (their influence may be passive, purely as a number, but this is nevertheless a power to be reckoned with in a regime of population-based, formula-driven resource allocation); the people who collect, code, store, transmit and order the data to be used in the calculation of the formula; the people who provide services to the people in the population, and whose work is recorded in the databases used to calculate the morbidity terms in funding formulas; the people who interrogate the databases and actually calculate the formula; and the people who participate in the discourse over the design of the formula. Any of these may be health policy activists. The activist's involvement is particularly concerned with orienting the formula to improving the operation of the health system for the benefit of the people served by it.

The effectiveness of the insider policy activist's involvement depends on understanding (perhaps in a statistical way) the makeup of the population, its health and health service use profile, and the characteristics and pressures in health services. It also depends on having an understanding of the institutional design of the health system. Knowledge across these fields underpins the relevance, technical acuity and political acceptability of proposals for formula design that emerge in the discourse. Health policy activists working in the field of resource distribution for health pride themselves on things such as their feel for the effects of various formula configurations on the population or a segment of it (e.g. see Ferrer 1993) and health service agencies, together with their capacity to recognise and articulate mechanisms that would produce valued changes to the health system. The insider activist's role is to connect the political objectives of the activist's cause—in health, this is more often than not to do with the pursuit of equity in one sense or another—with the administrative technologies available to govern the health system.

ACTIVIST AND INSTITUTION

The preceding few pages explored in turn the motivations, ethics, tasks and technologies of policy activism inside government agencies. Each has described to some extent the relationship between the insider activist and the institution, and an implicit common thread has been that this relationship constitutes and structures the subjective experience of insider activism. In this concluding section I take up this thread explicitly, and reflect on the way the experience of activism within government agencies challenges the identity of the activist as an institutional employee, and the identity of the institutional employee as an activist.

The starting point for this analysis is an understanding that institutions themselves display an ethics at the institutional level. How can this be so?

Public institutions have to frame an account of themselves—their *raison d'être* and their activities—in terms of specific public purposes that fit the portfolio with which they are engaged. It is these publicly oriented statements of mission, and their articulation within corporate documents, that provide an important domain for the work of the insider activist. This work includes the formulation of statements of the ethos of the institution, their publication, and the use of these statements to orient the programs of the institution.

By taking these statements at face value, and ensuring they do not stand as empty rhetoric, the insider policy activist can work towards the ethos of the institution being expressed in the policy discourse. Many health organisations openly acknowledge the importance of equity, excellence, effectiveness and efficiency as the ethos for what that organisation is trying to do. They may also guide the balance between various values—for example, between excellence and equity.

It is the internal relations of insider policy activists to the institution that determine the ethics of their activism and the components in the division of activist labour that they can most usefully pursue. At this point, a subtle question arises: is the insider activist acting as part of the institution, contributing to its ethos and through that contributing to its value for society, or operating as an activist against the institution? This is in some respects a question of strategy: which is the more successful strategy for positioning oneself as an activist? For people who are within the institution, it is important to be seen to be trying to promote it, in order to gain a better reception for their ideas by the other people in the institution. It also may enhance their capacity to access the institution's processes for the enunciation of policy and procedures for strategic planning.

The traditional perspective of the activist versus the system puts collaboration in terms of co-option: a selling out of the activist position in favour of working for the interests of the institution. This is a common concern for activists based in social movements (Papadakis 1984, Ch. 10). But by denying the possibility of ethical cooperation, and by refusing to appreciate that a change in the institutional ethos towards what is being promoted by the activist can give a legitimate advantage to the institution, this perspective cannot make sense of the actions of somebody trying to affect the institutional ethos from within.

In suggesting that activists can work positively within government agencies, I am not wanting to discount that at times the ethos of the institution may be virtually incompatible with the pursuit of any activist cause. Periodically, institutions become subject to intense efforts to reduce expenditure or restructure their internal organisation. During these periods, the institution may well be so functionally disabled that it cannot pursue its stated goals, much less respond to any activist agenda of relevance to the community it serves. Insider activists may cope with these periods by putting any activist projects on the back burner; advising community-based activists to not draw attention to any cause which could be detrimentally affected by the fiscal or structural agendas in play; or by leaving the organisation—a particularly attractive option for the activist professional who can return to community practice. All of these options may do little for the activist's sense of honour or commitment but, in short, survival skills must come into play. Intense periods of organisational change present the insider activist with risks and possibilities. They may do well or they may do badly. From personal observation I suspect that in times of organisational turmoil, junior insider activists tend to do well and senior insider activists tend to do poorly, whichever party is in government. In any case, the focus must shift from the immediate pursuit of activist causes to the security and structural location of the activist in the institution.

The need to survive to be useful, the importance of working with rather than against the institution, the ambiguities between activist and professional roles in the policy process, and the technical demands of the exercise of power all have implications for the sense of identity of the insider policy activist. This chapter has suggested that we try to understand policy activism inside government agencies as an immanent experience to which activists give themselves, a vocation to which they are called. On the one hand, the causes of such activism are rooted in community experience. On the other, the activity of the activist emerges immanently from their social location inside the agency. Because the experience of insider activism straddles this divide, the subjective position of the insider policy activist—constituted as it is by his or her internal relationship to the institution—rarely affords the comfort of feeling 'absolutely in accord with oneself'. The experience of insider activism requires a commitment to such experience, but may be ill-served by too firm an attachment to a specific cause or an overweening sense of righteousness.

The need to recognise a variety of causes and the capacity to cope with personal tensions and contradictions have implications for the ethics of insider activism: they work against the viability of a transcendental activist ethics and in favour of an immanent activism. It is an immanent, pragmatic ethics that determines the motivation of the activist to be on the lookout for opportunities within the activist discourse; that determines the value of policy know-how as an activist technology; and that allows us to recognise—as did my friend from student politics days—that for the activist, working within government agencies can be an intensifier of thought and a multiplier of the forms and domains for political action.

Policy-making is always in part obscure. Even if there is an ethos of open government—increasingly rare in government agencies, it seems—some secrecy and some impenetrable complexity will always remain part of life for policy workers. This makes it important that people working in policy, especially those with an activist bent, take the trouble to open their thinking to the community. The common experience of explaining a policy rationale to people who do not want to understand it can make policy workers reticent to explain what they do outside of the work environment, but public-spiritedness and intellectual generosity will in general overcome this. As well as sharpening one's analysis, writing, teaching, speaking at conferences, taking on cadets and interns, even a well-judged discussion with friends, can all help to increase the community's understanding of policy work. It is an interesting line of work.

BIBLIOGRAPHY

AGB Australia 1992a, 'GP choice I: A qualitative investigation of customer attitudes towards GP systems', unpublished research report, AGB Australia, Sydney.

—— 1992b, 'GP choice II: A qualitative investigation of GPs' attitudes towards GP systems', unpublished research report, AGB Australia, Sydney.

—— 1992c, 'Patients' choice of general practitioner: Quantitative report', unpublished research report, AGB Australia, Sydney.

Aldrich, R. 2006, 'Flesh-coloured bandaids: Politics, discourse policy and the health of Aboriginal and Torres Strait Islander Peoples 1972–2001', unpublished PhD thesis, University of New South Wales, Sydney.

Alfred, T. 2005, *Wasase: Indigenous pathways of action and freedom*, Broadview Press, Perterborough, ON, Canada.

Allan, B. 1987, *FMIP and program budgeting: A study of implementation in selected agencies*, AGPS, Canberra.

Altman, D. 1988, *A politics of poetry: Reconstituting social democracy*, Pluto Press, Sydney.

Andersen, T.F. and Mooney, G. (eds) 1990, *The challenges of medical practice variation*, Macmillan, London.

Anderson, I. 2007, 'The policy process', in B. Carson, T. Dunbar, R.D. Chenhall and R. Bailie (eds), *Social determinants of Indigenous health*, Allen & Unwin, Sydney.

Appleby, J. 1992, *Financing health care in the 1990s*, Open University Press, Buckingham.

Arabena, K. 2005, *Not fit for modern society: Aboriginal and Torres Strait Islander people and the new arrangements for the administration of Indigenous affairs*, AIATSIS, Canberra.

Arrow, K.J. 1963, 'Uncertainty and the welfare economics of medical care', *American Economic Review*, vol. 53, pp. 941–73.

Australian Community Health Association (ACHA) 1986, *Review of the community health program*, Redfern Legal Centre Publishing, Sydney.

Australian Government Solicitor 1993, *Agreement between the Commonwealth of Australia and the State of New South Wales in relation to the provision of public hospital services and other health services from 1 July 1993 to 30 June 1998 under section 24 of the Health Insurance Act 1973 (Cth)*, Australian Government Solicitor, Canberra.

Australian Health Ministers Advisory Committee (AHMAC) Breast Cancer Screening Evaluation Committee 1990, *Breast cancer screening in Australia: Future directions*, AGPS, Canberra.

Australian Health Ministers Advisory Committee (AHMAC) Health Targets and Implementation Committee 1988, *Health for all Australians*, AGPS, Canberra.

Australian Institute of Health and Welfare (AIHW) 1994, *Australia's health 1994*, AGPS, Canberra.

—— 2006, *Australia's health 2006*, AGPS, Canberra.

Bailey, P., Lightly, E. and Rimmer, J. 1978, *Consultative arrangements and the co-ordination of social policy development*, AGPS, Canberra.

Barr, E.L.M., Magliano, D.J., Zimmet, P.Z. et al. 2006, *AusDiab 2005: The Australian diabetes, obesity and lifestyle study. Tracking the accelerating epidemic: its causes and outcomes*, International Diabetes Institute, Melbourne.

Barre-Sinoussi, F. et al. 1983, 'Isolation of a T-Lymphatropic retrovirus from a patient at risk for acquired immune deficiency syndrome (AIDS)', *Science*, vol. 220, no. 4599, pp. 868–71.

Baume, P.E. 1994, *A cutting edge: Australia's surgical workforce*, Commonwealth Department of Health, Housing, Local Government and Community Services, Canberra.

Beck, U. 1992, *Risk society: Toward a new modernity*, Sage, London.

Beiner, R. (ed.) 1995, *Theorising citizenship*, State University of New York Press, New York.

Bell, E.T. 1953, *Men of mathematics*, Penguin, Harmondsworth.

Berlin, I. 1969, *Four essays on liberty*, Oxford University Press, London.

Berry, T. 1999, *The great work: Our way into the future*, Random House, New York.

Beveridge, W.H. 1942, *Social insurance and allied services: report* [Beveridge report], Macmillan, New York.

Bierce, A. 1967, *The enlarged devil's dictionary*, Penguin, Harmondsworth.

Blomquist, A.G. and Carter, R.A.L. 1995, 'Is health care really a luxury?', seminar paper presented at the Department of Economics, University of Western Ontario.

Boorse, C. 1977, 'Health as a theoretical concept', *Philosophy of Science*, vol. 44, pp. 542–73.

Boston, J. (ed.) 1995, *The state under contract*, Bridget Williams Books, Wellington.

Braithwaite, J. 1993a, 'Identifying the elements in the Australian health service management revolution', *Australian Journal of Public Affairs*, vol. 52, no. 4, pp. 417–30.

—— 1993b, 'Strategic management and organisational structure: Transformation process at work in hospitals', *Australian Health Review*, vol. 14, no. 4, pp. 383–405.

Braithwaite, J. and Drahos, P. 2000, *Global business regulation*, Cambridge University Press, Cambridge.

Braithwaite, J., Makkai, T. and Braithwaite, V. (2007), *Regulating aged care: ritualism and the new pyramid*, Edward Elger, Cheltenham.

Broom, D.H. 1991, *Speaking for themselves: Consumer issues in the restructuring of general practice*, NCEPH discussion paper no. 4, NCEPH, Australian National University, Canberra.

Burchell, G. 1993, 'Liberal government and techniques of the self', *Economy and Society*, vol. 22, pp. 267–82.

Burchell, G., Gordon, C. and Miller, P. (eds) 1991, *The Foucault effect: Studies in governmentality with two lectures and an interview with Michel Foucault*, Harvester Wheatsheaf, London.

Butler, J.R.G. 1994, 'How do economists see the world?', in *General Practice Evaluation Program of Commonwealth Department of Human Services & Health Quality and Value: 1994 Work-in-progress conference proceedings*, GPEP, DHS&H, Canberra, pp. 19–40.

Carson, B., Dunbar, T., Chenhall, R.D. and Bailie, R. 2007, *Social determinants of Indigenous health*, Allen & Unwin, Sydney.

Chaudhuri, A. 2004, 'In the waiting room of history', *London Review of Books*, June.

Clapham, K., O'Dea, K. and Chenhall, R. 2007, 'Interventions and sustainable programs', in B. Carson, T. Dunbar, R.D. Chenhall and R. Bailie (eds), *Social determinants of Indigenous health*, Allen & Unwin, Sydney.

Commonwealth Department of Community Services and Health (DCSH) 1989a, *Commonwealth Department of Community Services and Health National Women's Health Policy: Advancing women's health in Australia*, AGPS Canberra.

—— 1989b, *Annual report 1988–89*, AGPS, Canberra.

Commonwealth Department of Health (CDH) 1984, *Annual report 1983–84*, AGPS, Canberra.

Commonwealth Department of Health, Housing, Local Government and Community Services (DHHLG&CS) 1993, *Annual report 1992–93*, AGPS, Canberra.

Commonwealth Department of Human Services and Health 1995, *Continuity of care, quality and the Better Practice Program*, Commonwealth Department of Human Services and Health, Canberra.

Commonwealth of Australia 1989, *National HIV/AIDS strategy: A policy information paper* [White paper], AGPS, Canberra.

Considine, M. and Painter, M. 1997, *Managerialism: The great debate*, Melbourne University Press, Melbourne.

Coombs, H.C. 1976, *Report of the Royal Commission on Australian Government Administration*, AGPS, Canberra.

Cooper, M.H. and Culyer, A.J. 1973, *Health economics: Selected readings*, Penguin, Harmondsworth.

Costello, P. and Fahey, J. 1996, *Budget Paper No. 2*, Government Printer, Canberra.

Cumming, R.G., Barton, G.E. et al. 1989, 'Medical practitioners and health promotion: Results from a survey in Sydney's Western Suburbs', *Community Health Studies*, vol. 13, no. 3, pp. 294–300.

Daniel, A. 1990, *Medicine and the state*, Allen & Unwin, Sydney.

Davis, G., Sullivan, B. and Yeatman, A. 1996, *A new contractualism?*, Macmillan, Melbourne.

Davis, G., Wanna, J., Warhurst, J. and Weller, P. 1993, *Public policy in Australia* (2nd edn), Allen & Unwin, Sydney.

Dean, M. 1991, *The constitution of poverty: Toward a genealogy of liberal governance*, Routledge, London.

Defert, D. 1991, '"Popular life" and insurance technology', in G. Burchell, C. Gordon and P. Miller (eds), *The Foucault effect*, Harvester Wheatsheaf, London, pp. 211–34.

Deloria, V. 1968, *Custer died for your sins: An Indian manifesto*, University of Oklahoma Press, Norman.

Dodson, M. 2007, *Mabo speech*, AIATSIS, Canberra.

Doherty, P. 1988, *Australian medical education and workforce into the 21st century*, Commonwealth Department of Community Services and Health, Canberra.

Douglas, R.M. (ed.) 1991, *General practice financing think tank: Proceedings of a meeting of general practitioners, economists, social scientists and administrators*, NCEPH, Australian National University, Canberra.

Douglas, R.M. and Saltman, D.C. (eds) 1991, *W(h)ither Australian general practice?*, NCEPH discussion paper no. 1, Australian National University, Canberra.

Drummond, M.F. 1980, *Principles of economic appraisal in health care*, Oxford University Press, Oxford.

Duckett, S.J. 2004, *The Australian health system* (2nd edn), Oxford University Press, Melbourne.

Dugdale, P. 1991, 'The management of consumer advocacy', *Australian Journal of Public Administration*, vol. 50, no. 1, pp. 17–22.

—— 1992a, 'Public management in the welfare state. Managerialism and consumer advocacy in the 1980s', MA thesis, Australian National University.

—— 1992b, 'Review of *The price of health* by James Gillespie', *Current Affairs Bulletin*, vol. 68, no. 9, pp. 29–30.

—— 1994, 'Review of *Health financing in the 1990s* by John Appleby', *Australian Journal of Public Health*, vol. 18, no. 3, pp. 346–8.

—— 1998, 'The art of insider activism: Policy activism and the governance of health', in A. Yeatman (ed.), *Activism and the policy process*, Allen & Unwin, Sydney.

—— 2007, 'Influenza vaccination for healthy adults', *Australian Prescriber*, April.

Dugdale, P. and Kelsall, L. 2004, *ACT Chief Health Officer's Report 2000–2002*, ACT Health, Canberra.

Ellwood, P.M. 1988, 'Outcomes management: A technology of patient experience' (Shattuck Lecture), *New England Journal of Medicine*, vol. 318, no. 23, pp. 1549–56.

Ewald, F. 1991, 'Insurance and risk', in G. Burchell, C. Gordon and P. Miller (eds), *The Foucault effect*, Harvester Wheatsheaf, London, pp. 197–210.

Ferrer, E. 1993, 'Resource allocation models in health: Implications for the provision of services to people from non-English speaking backgrounds', paper delivered at the Health for Multicultural Australia National Conference, Sydney.

Flew, A. 1970, 'Introduction', in T. Malthus, *An essay on the principle of population*, Penguin, Harmondsworth.

—— 1979, *A dictionary of philosophy*, Pan, London.

Foucault M. 1971, *Madness and civilisation: A history of insanity in the age of reason*, Tavistock, London.

—— 1972, *The archaeology of knowledge and the discourse on language*, Pantheon, New York.

—— 1973, *The birth of the clinic: An archaeology of medical perception*, Tavistock, London.

—— 1976, *History of sexuality, vol. 1*, Penguin, Harmondsworth.

—— 1977, *Discipline and punish: The birth of the prison*, Penguin, Harmondsworth.

—— 1980, *Power/knowledge: Selected interviews and other writings by Michel Foucault* (ed. C. Gordon), Harvester Wheatsheaf, London.

—— 1983, Preface, in G. Deleuze and F. Guattari (eds) 1983, *Anti-Oedipus: Capitalism and schizophrenia*, University of Minnesota Press, Minneapolis.

—— 1986, *The use of pleasure: The history of sexuality, vol. 2*, Vintage Books, New York.

—— 1988, *The care of the self: The history of sexuality, vol. 3*, Vintage Books, New York.

—— 1990a [1970], *The order of things*, Tavistock, London.

—— 1990b [1980], 'The politics of health in the eighteenth century', in M. Foucault, *The order of things*, Vintage Books, London.

—— 1991, 'Governmentality', in G. Burchell, C. Gordon and P. Miller (eds), *The Foucault effect*, Harvester Wheatsheaf, London, pp. 87–104.

—— 1997 *Ethics, subjectivity and truth*, New Press, New York.

Freebairn, L. 2007, *The health of the Aboriginal and Torres Strait Islander people in the ACT*, ACT Health, Canberra.

Friedman, F. and Friedman, R.D. 1980, *Free to choose*, Penguin, Harmondsworth.

Gadamer, H.G. 1996, *The enigma of health: The art of healing in a scientific age*, Stanford University Press, Stanford.

Gane, M. and Johnson, T. 1993, *Foucault's new domains*, Routledge, London.

General Practice Consultative Committee (GPCC) 1992, *The future of general practice: A strategy for the nineties and beyond*, AMA/RACGP/Commonwealth Department of Health, Housing and Community Services, Canberra.

Gillespie, J.A. 1991, *The price of health: Australian governments and medical politics 1910–1960*, Cambridge University Press, Melbourne.

Gordon, C. 1991, 'Governmental rationality: An introduction', in G. Burchell, C. Gordon and P. Miller (eds), *The Foucault effect*, Harvester Wheatsheaf, London, pp. 1–52.

Habermas, J., Derrida, J. and Borradori, G. 2003, *Philosophy in a time of terror: Dialogues with Jurgen Habermas and Jacques Derrida*, University of Chicago Press, Chicago.

Hacking, I. 1990, *The taming of chance*, Cambridge University Press, Cambridge.

Ham, C. 2004, *Health policy in Britain* (5th edn), Palgrave, Basingstoke.

Harris, L. 1994, 'Funding and general practice quality', in *General Practice Evaluation Program of Commonwealth Department of Human Services and Health Quality and Value: Work-in-progress conference proceedings*, GPEP, Canberra, pp. 69–76.

Hayek, F.A. 1944, *The road to serfdom*, Routledge and Kegan Paul, London.

Herzlich, C. 1973, *Health and illness*, Academic Press, London.

Hindess, B. 1987, *Freedom, equality and the market: Arguments on social policy*, Tavistock, London.

—— 1996, *Discourses of power: From Hobbes to Foucault*, Polity, London.

Holland, W.W., Detels, R. and Knox, G. 1991, *Oxford textbook of public health* (2nd edn), Oxford University Press, London.

Holy Bible 1989, New Revised Standard Edition, John 18:38, Thomas Nelson, Nashville.

Howard, J. 2005, 'Transcript of Australia Day Flag-raising Ceremony', Office of the Prime Minister, Canberra.

Human Rights and Equal Opportunity Commission (HREOC) 1997, *Bringing them home: Report of the National Inquiry into the Separation of Aboriginal and Torres Strait Islander Children from Their Families*, Commonwealth of Australia, Canberra.

Ibsen, H. 1981, *Hedda Gabler*, in H. Ibsen, *Four Major Plays*, Oxford University Press, London.

Industry Commission 1997, *Private Health Insurance*, AGPS, Canberra.

International Monetary Fund (IMF) 2001, *Government finance statistics manual*, IMF, Paris.

James, B.C. 2005, *Quality management for health care delivery, health research and education trust*, Chicago.

Jamison, J.H. 1980, *Commission of Inquiry into the Efficiency and Administration of Hospitals*, 3 vols, AGPS, Canberra.

Jeffs, D. 1994, 'More about that pump handle', *Snow's Field: Newsletter of the AFPHM*, vol. 4, no. 3, p. 8.

Jenkinson, C. (ed.) 1994, *Measuring health and medical outcomes*, University College London.

Johnston, E. 1991, *Royal Commission into Aboriginal Deaths in Custody: National report*, Commonwealth of Australia, Canberra.

Journal of Health Services 2004, *Research Supplement*, October, Blackwell, London.

Keane, J. 2004, *Violence and democracy*, Cambridge University Press, Cambridge.

Keating, M. 1988, 'Managing for results: The challenge for finance and agencies', *Canberra Bulletin of Public Administration*, March, pp. 73–80.

—— 1989, 'Quo vadis? Challenges of public administration', *Australian Journal of Public Administration*, vol. 48, no. 2.

Keith, A. 1994, 'Renegotiation of the Medicare Agreement: Some reflections on the policy process', seminar presentation, NCEPH, Australian National University, Canberra.

Kunitz, S.J. 1996, *Disease and social diversity: The European impact on the health of non-Europeans*, Oxford University Press, New York.

Lane, R. 2000, *The loss of happiness in market democracies*, Yale University Press, New Haven, CN.

Laszlo, E. 2004, *Science and the Akashic field: An integral theory of everything* (2nd edn), Inner Traditions, Rochester.

Latour, B. 1988, *The Pasteurization of France*, Harvard University Press, Cambridge, MA.

Lewis, J. 1991, 'Origins and development of public health in the UK', in W.W. Holland, R. Detels and G. Knox, *Oxford textbook of public health* (2nd edn), Oxford University Press, London.

Lindblom, C.E. 1977, *Politics and markets: The world's political-economic systems*, Basic Books, New York.

Lloyd, P. 1994, 'A history of medical professionalisation in NSW: 1788–1950', *Australian Health Review*, vol. 17, no. 2.

Macklin, J. 1991, *Hospital services in Australia: Access and financing*, National Health Strategy Issues Paper No. 2, Commonwealth Department of Health, Housing and Community Services, Canberra.

—— 1992, *The future of general practice*, National Health Strategy Issues Paper No. 3, Commonwealth Department of Health, Housing and Community Services, Canberra.

Malthus, T. 1970 [1798], *An essay on the principle of population* (ed. A. Flew), Penguin, Harmondsworth.

Marano, N., Arguin, P., Pappaioanou, M. and King, L. 2005, 'Role of multisector partnerships in controlling emerging zoonotic diseases', *Emerging Infectious Diseases*, vol. 11, no. 12, pp. 1–6.

Markel, H. 2004, '"I swear by Apollo": On taking the Hippocratic Oath', *New England Journal of Medicine*, vol. 350, no. 20, pp. 2026–9.

Marmot, M. 2004, *Status syndrome: How your social standing directly affects your health and life expectancy*, Bloomsbury, London, 2004.

Mason, Brennan, Deane, Dawson, Toohey, Gaudron and Mchugh JJ 1992, *Mabo v Queensland*, High Court of Australia, Canberra.

McCallum, J., Raymond, C. and McGilchrist, C. 1995, 'Patient continuity of care: patient and practice effects', personal communication of unpublished draft, February 1995, NCEPH, Australian National University, Canberra.

McGuire, A., Henderson, J. and Mooney, G.H. 1988, *The economics of health care: An introductory text*, RKP, London.

McMichael, A.J. 2006, 'Population health as the "bottom line" of sustainability: A contemporary challenge for public health researchers', *European Journal of Public Health*, vol. 16, no. 6, pp. 579–81.

Medicare Australia 2006, *Annual report 2005–06*, Australian Government, Canberra.

Miettinen, O.S. 1985, *Theoretical epidemiology: Principles of occurrence research in medicine*, John Wiley & Sons, New York.

Mooney, G.H. 1986, *Economics, medicine and health care*, Harvester Wheatsheaf, London.

Moore, K.L. 1977, *The developing human: Clinically oriented embryology* (2nd edn), W.B. Saunders, Washington.

Muecke, S. 2004, *Ancient and modern: Time, culture and Indigenous philosophy*, University of New South Wales Press, Sydney.

Nakata, M. 2007, *Disciplining the savages, savaging the disciplines*, Aboriginal Studies Press, Canberra.

National Centre for Classification in Health (NCCH) 1997, *ICD–10-AM implementation kit*, NCCH, University of Sydney.

National Health and Medical Research Council 2004, *Australian drinking water guidelines*, NHMRC, Canberra.

National Specialist Qualification Advisory Committee of Australia (NSQAC) 1995, *Recommended medical specialties and qualifications No. 23*, Commonwealth of Australia, Canberra.

Nietzsche, F. 1966 [1886], *Beyond good and evil: Prelude to a philosophy of the future*, Vintage, New York.

—— 1969 [1887], *On the genealogy of morals* (trans. W. Kaufmann), Random House, New York.

NSW Government 1995a, *Economic statement for health*, NSW Health Department, Sydney.

—— 1995b, *Caring for health: Equity efficiency and quality*, NSW Government Economic Statement for Health, NSW Health Department, Sydney.

NSW Health 2005, *NSW Health's funding approach*, NSW Health, Sydney.

NSW Health Department 1990, *A resource allocation formula for the NSW health system*, NSW Health Department, Sydney.

—— 1991a, *A discussion paper on health outcomes*, NSW Health Department, Sydney.

—— 1991b, *Changing the shape of the NSW health system*, NSW Health Department, Sydney.

—— 1992, *The NSW Health Outcomes Initiative discussion paper*, NSW Health Department, Sydney.

—— 1993, *Leading the way: A framework for NSW mental health services 1991–2001*, NSW Health Department, Sydney.

—— 1994, *Getting it right: Focusing on the outcomes of health services and programs*, NSW Health Department, Sydney.

—— 1996a, *NSW area strategic planning guidelines for budget allocation, achievements of benchmark costs and cross boundary purchasing*, NSW Health Department, Sydney.

—— 1996b, *Implementation of the Economic Statement for Health*, NSW Health Department, Sydney.

—— 1996c, *Implementation of the economic statement for health*, NSW Health Department, Sydney.

Offe, C. 1984, *Contradictions of the welfare state*, Century Hutchinson, London.

Opit, L.J. 1984, 'The cost of health care and health insurance in Australia: Some problems associated with the fee for service system', *Social Science & Medicine*, vol. 18, pp. 967–72.

Osborne, T. 1993, 'On the "liberal profession" of medicine', *Economy and Society*, vol. 22, pp. 345–56.

Palmer, G.R. and Short, S.D. 2000, *Health care and public policy: An Australian analysis* (3rd edn), Macmillan, Melbourne.

Papadakis, E. 1984, *The Green movement in West Germany*, Croom Helm, London.

Papadakis, E. and Taylor-Gooby, P. 1987, *The private provision of public welfare: State, market and community*, Wheatsheaf, Sussex.

Parsons, T. 1952, *The social system*, RKP, London.

Penman, R. and Dugdale, P. 2003, *Quality and safety in ACT health care: Report on progress*, ACT Health, Canberra.

Pensabene, T.S. 1980, *The rise of the medical profession in Victoria*, Health Research Project, ANU, Canberra.

Phillips, C.B., Patel, M.S., Glasgow, N., Pearce, C., Dugdale, P., Davies, A., Hall, S. and Kljakovic, M. 2007, 'Australian general practice and pandemic influenza: Models of clinical practice in an established pandemic', *Medical Journal of Australia*, vol. 186, pp. 355–8.

Prevost, J.A., Carr, M.P. and Dilley, J.W. 1992, 'A round table discussion: hospital leaders discuss QI implementation issues', *Quality Review Bulletin*, March.

Public Health Association of Australia 1997, *Policies of the Public Health Association*, PHA, Canberra.

Pusey, M. 1991, *Economic rationalism in Canberra*, Cambridge University Press, Sydney.

Ridgeway, A. 2005, 'A valedictory speech to the Australian Senate, 22 June 2005', Australian Parliamentary *Hansard*, quoted in R. Aldrich (2006), 'Flesh-coloured bandaids: Politics, discourse policy and the health of Aboriginal and Torres Strait Islander Peoples 1972–2001', unpublished PhD thesis, University of New South Wales, Sydney.

Rivers, W.H.R. 2001 [1924], *Medicine, magic and religion: The Fitzpatrick Lectures delivered before the Royal College of Physicians of London in 1915 and 1916*, Routledge, London.

Rizaz, F. 2003, 'SARS virus identified by scientists', *Johns Hopkins News-Letter*, 4 April.

Rose, N. 1989, *Governing the soul*, Routledge, London.

—— 1992, *Towards a critical sociology of freedom: Inaugural lecture*, Goldsmith's College, University of London.

—— 1993, 'Government, authority and expertise in advanced liberalism', *Economy and society*, vol. 22, pp. 283–99.

Rose, N. and Miller, P. 1992, 'Political power beyond the state: Problematics of government', *British Journal of Sociology*, vol. 43, pp. 173–205.

Rosenman, S.J. and Mackinnon, A. 1992, 'General practitioner services under Medicare', *Australian Journal of Public Health*, vol. 16, no. 4, pp. 419–26.

Rowse, T. 1998, *White flour, white power: From rations to citizenship in Central Australia*, Cambridge University Press, New York.

Royal Australian College of General Practitioners (RACGP) 1993, *Entry standards for general practice accreditation: Draft standards for field testing and trials*, RACGP, Sydney.

Runciman, W.G. 1978, 'Preface', in M. Weber, *Selections in translation* (ed. W.G. Runciman), Cambridge University Press, Cambridge.

Russell, B. 1979, *History of western philosophy*, Allen & Unwin, London.

Sanders, W. 2007, 'Changes to CDEP under DWER: Policy substance and the new contractualism', *Impact: News Quarterly of ACOSS*, Autumn, pp. 6–7.

Saul, J.R. 2005, *Good governance as the key to Gross National Happiness: Proceedings of the 2nd International conference on gross national happiness*, Antigonish, Nova Scotia.

Sax, S. 1974, *Hospitals in Australia*, Report of the Hospital and Health Services Commission (H&HSC), H&HSC, Canberra.

—— 1984, *A strife of interests*, Allen & Unwin, Sydney.

Schwartz, C. (ed.) 1991, *Chambers concise dictionary*, Chambers, Edinburgh.

Scotton, R.B. and MacDonald, C.R. 1993, *The making of Medibank*, School of Health Services Management, University of NSW, Sydney.

Shaw, C., Fahey, P.P. and Ryan, S. 1991, *Continuous quality improvement: Engineering health care excellence*, Technical Report, Department of Statistics, University of Newcastle.

Sissons, J. 2005, *First peoples: Indigenous cultures and their futures*, Reaktion, London.

Soya, E. 1996, *Thirdspace: Journeys to Los Angeles and other real and imagined places*, Blackwell, London.

Taylor, G.F. 1911, *Principles of scientific management*, Harper, New York.

Tortora, G.J., Funke, B.R. and Case, C.L. 1995, *Microbiology: An introduction* (5th edn), Benjamin/Cummings, Redwood City.

Turner, B. 1987, *Medical knowledge and social power*, Sage, London.

Uhr, J. 1987, 'Towards resourceful public administration: A management polemic', *Australian Journal of Public Administration*, vol. 46, no. 4.

United Kingdom Department of Health 1989, *Working for patients* [white paper], HMSO, London.

United Nations 2006, *Declaration on the Rights of Indigenous Peoples*, United Nations, New York.

United Nations International Children's Emergency Fund (UNICEF) 1999, *Child and Maternal Mortality Survey*, UNICEF, New York.

United States Centre for Disease Control 1981, *Morbidity and mortality weekly report*, 18 June.

Vanstone, A. 2005, quoted in *The Australian*, 21 November, p. 1.

Veale, B.M. and Douglas, R.M. 1992, *Money matters in general practice financing options and restructuring*, NCEPH discussion paper no. 6, Australian National University, Canberra.

Weber, M. 1978a, *Selections in translation* (ed. W.G. Runciman), Cambridge University Press, Cambridge.

—— 1978b [1919], 'Politics as a vocation', in *Selections in translation* (ed. W.G. Runciman), Cambridge University Press, Cambridge, pp. 212–25.

White, K. 1999, 'Negotiating science and liberalism: Medicine in nineteenth century South Australia', *Medical History*, vol. 43, pp. 173–91.

Wildavsky, A. 1979, *The politics of the budgetary process*, Little, Brown, Boston.

Wilenski, P. 1982, *Unfinished agenda: Further report of the Review of NSW government administration*, NSW Government, Sydney.

—— 1988, 'Social change as a source of competing values in public administration', *Australian Journal of Public Administration*, vol. 47, no. 3.

Wilkinson, R. and Marmot, M. 2003, *Social determinants of health: the solid facts*, WHO, Geneva.

Williams, R. 1992, *Remission impossible: The future of the Australian health industry*, Jacaranda, Brisbane.

Willis, E. 1983, *Medical dominance*, George Allen & Unwin, Sydney.

Wooldridge, M. 1991, Health policy in the Fraser years, 1975–1983, unpublished MBA thesis, Monash University, Melbourne.

Wootton, B. 1945, *Freedom under planning*, Allen & Unwin, London.

World Health Organization (WHO) 1946, *Constitution of the World Health Organization*, WHO, Geneva.

—— 1986, 'Ottawa Charter for Health Promotion', *Canadian Journal of Public Health*, vol. 77, pp. 425–30.

—— 1992, *International statistical classification of diseases and related health problems—tenth revision* (ICD-IO), WHO, Geneva.

—— 2004a, 'Avian influenza A(H5N1) in humans and poultry in Viet Nam', *WHO Disease Outbreak News*, 13 January.

—— 2004b, *Guidelines for the global surveillance of Severe Acute Respiratory Syndrome (SARS): Updated recommendations*, WHO, Geneva, October.

Yeatman, A. 1990a, *Bureaucrats, technocrats, femocrats: Essays on the contemporary Australian state*, Allen & Unwin, Sydney.

—— 1990b, 'Reconstructing public bureaucracies: The residualisation of equity and access', *Australian Journal of Public Administration*, vol. 49, no. 1.

—— 1995, 'Interpreting contemporary contractualism', in J. Boston (ed.), *The state under contract*, Bridget Williams Books, Wellington.

—— 1996, *Getting real: The final report of the review of the Commonwealth/State Disability Agreement*, AGPS, Canberra.

—— (ed.) 1998, *Activism and the policy process*, Allen & Unwin, Sydney.

Youngson, A.J. 1979, *The scientific revolution in Victorian medicine*, ANU Press, Canberra.

INDEX

Printed in the United States
by Baker & Taylor Publisher Services